Everything You Ever Wanted to Know About the Back

Everything You Ever Wanted to Know About the Back

A consumers guide to the diagnosis
and treatment of lower back pain

Donald Steven Corenman, M.D., D.C

www.neckandback.com

To order additional copies of this book, contact:
Xlibris Corporation
1-888-795-4274
www.Xlibris.com
Orders@Xlibris.com
48706

Contents

Kim, Jessica, Steven and Samantha—
Thank you for your wonderful support and love.

To Charmayne Bernhardt, thanks for your artistic talent.

Introduction

Why another book on lower back and leg pain? Well, lower back pain is the second most common reason to visit a doctor, right behind colds and the flu. Low back pain costs American society 50 billion dollars a year. With regard to productivity, it is the most costly problem in the industrial world. Eighty percent of the population will have disabling back pain at one time in their lives.

The irony is that in medical school, there is little or no time spent with the education of medical students regarding the causes and treatment of lower back disorders. Chiropractic schools and physical therapy schools have more emphasis on this subject, but the information presented can be sketchy and incomplete. Considering the dearth of knowledge on this subject, it seemed that a book was warranted.

Go to Amazon.com, and you can find more than one hundred titles regarding how to diagnose and cure the back. Some are accurate, and some have significant misinformation. Many nonacademic texts always seem to boil down to the "fact" that there is no real way to fully understand the causes of back or leg pain and give a standard treatment protocol for all spine problems. This concept is simply incorrect. Almost all pain and dysfunction that the spine generates can be diagnosed and treated. The academic texts, even though complete, are so difficult to understand and interpret that for many, they seem to be written in Chinese.

The style of this book is repetition. If you are a spine surgeon, boredom will set in quickly. However, if you are a pain sufferer or a nonspine health care professional, the repetition will be helpful to instill the understanding of this "new language."

I have been involved with spine for thirty years, and my thinking processes are pretty straightforward. I have simplified many of the concepts of anatomy, physiology, and pathology so that I can personally understand and use them on a daily basis. Since I had to break things down into small logical bites for myself, I thought it might be worthwhile to write it all down for others to use. Using this book, whether you are a caregiver or a patient, will allow you to understand and master this subject and take the mystery out of the spine.

This text is not, however, a cookbook. Reading this book will give you a reasonable understanding of why problems occur and how to treat them, but not the specifics of how many repetitions of what exercises to do. This tome will allow you to know which exercises may be of benefit and which ones could be harmful. It won't tell you when you need surgery but will allow you to question those practitioners as to the right direction to go. This book will tell you how to find the right professional and double-check the information they convey.

For patients, the straightforward knowledge of why you may have pain that will not put you in a wheelchair or paralyze you may be enough to keep from worrying about your back. If that is not enough, this book will give you some tools to treat your back or find the right caregiver to help you.

I have no doubt that some spine-care experts may read this book and have problems with the liberties I have taken to simplify these subjects. Making a complex subject easy to understand requires some shortcuts and poetic license. I hope I haven't offended anyone, but I have put on my flame suit. I do believe this book is accurate and accessible.

The knowledge of the spine chemically and mechanically is expanding at a great pace. Spine care may be significantly different ten years from now as it has changed in the last ten years. This book will need to be edited significantly in the years to come.

Personal History

So where do I come from, and why do I find myself writing this book? I didn't start my life with the intent to become a spine expert. My life circumstances have led me serendipitously into this field. I started out twenty-five years ago not knowing what to do in life. My cousin became a chiropractor, and I thought it would be interesting; so after college, I applied to the Los Angeles College of Chiropractic. I was promptly rejected, which started my competitive juices flowing. Being somewhat stubborn, I decided to help them change their minds. After some convincing, they agreed to let me in. Four uneventful years later, I had my degree in hand and attempted to heal the injured.

Well, I helped some patients but didn't help others. The reasons why I was successful at treating patients were very murky. My understanding of spine was incomplete. So I decided to take a residency in chiropractic orthopaedics. This was actually about three years of weekend education while I was still practicing standard chiropractic (I never understood why it wasn't called chiropractry). My knowledge base grew, but I was still unsatisfied with some of my results and all of my wisdom.

I then made the decision to go to medical school. I thought that after four more years of education, I finally would have a mastery of spine and the human body. Convincing a medical school that a chiropractor should be educated in the allopathic (traditional) model was a much greater challenge than getting into chiropractic school. After some interesting travels and experiences, Wayne State University in Michigan accepted me (bless their hearts).

As you can see, at the time, forethought of planning was not my strength. I failed to take into consideration that after medical school, there is still a five-year orthopaedic residency and then a one-year spinal disorders fellowship to consider. Ten years after starting with medical school, I was finally finished (or so I thought).

It took me three more years after being on staff at the University of Colorado lecturing and teaching residents and fellows to put my experience into perspective and to understand how the two disparate fields I learned were complementary and synergistic. Finally, the experience at the Steadman Hawkins Clinic has been very fulfilling to allow me to mature to this point. I continue to think I have finally "put it all together," but I still learn many new pearls every day.

Thanks to Dr. Richard Stonebrink, Dr. Maurice Castle, Dr. Tom Lowe, and Dr. Tony Dwyer for the great experience and education. Special thanks to Dr. Richard Steadman and my partners for allowing me to join the clinic. Eric Strauch, PAC, and

I have been partners for years, and he is invaluable. He should have gone to medical school as he could teach spine. He helps much in checking my knowledge. My staff of Margaret, Cheri, Diana, Vangie and Sara has been phenomenal. I owe much to all my prior teachers and professors. A big thank you to the residents, fellows, medical students, physician assistants, chiropractors, athletic trainers, and physical therapists that were very bright and asked very challenging questions. Finally, to all my patients who had enough faith in me to allow me to attempt and succeed in their treatment, thank you for all your patience (no pun intended).

1

The Basics

The successful diagnosis and treatment of spinal disorders is defined by the education and experience of the examiner. The root factor is a correct understanding of the diagnosis and what can be done to manage or cure the disorder. There is almost always an answer to a spinal problem. A majority of the time, management is the key. Management can include home exercises, activity avoidance, guided physical therapy program, chiropractic, medications, and ergonomics. Sometimes surgery can be an option or rarely mandatory.

The natural history of the disorder is important to know. That is, what would the malady do if left untreated? Spinal pain can be self-limiting, meaning it would go away if left on its own. If you didn't know this and had a practitioner treat the pain, the pain would disappear. Was it the treatment or just the passing of time that caused the success? Voltaire said, "The purpose of the doctor is to entertain the patient while nature affects the cure." In this case, treatment would simply be entertainment.

A good example is muscle overuse syndrome or muscle strain where the muscles become internally disorganized. The relationships between the internal proteins that cause muscle contraction become disassociated. This muscle soreness lasts two to three days and will resolve if left on its own. Of course, a good massage will improve symptoms and may limit the period of soreness by a day, but will not change the ultimate outcome. Medications will also reduce symptoms but won't change the eventual result. Knowing the diagnosis will lead to the appropriate therapy. There may not be a pressing need for treatment.

There are pains generated by the lower back that are significant and sometimes severe, but most of the time, low back pain is not dangerous. Many patients are fearful of paralysis and equate severe lower back pain with the eventual use of a wheelchair. This is simply not true for the vast majority of back pain. The proper diagnosis provides peace of mind and relieves anguish.

There are three foundations to make an appropriate diagnosis: history, physical examination, and confirmatory tests.

The history is probably the most important of the three foundations. The history is simply what happened to cause the symptoms, a list of the symptoms, and what activities and time of day make the symptoms better or worse. The activities and positions that aggravate the pain help to indicate the biomechanics of the disorder. The history will also include knowledge of other problems patients may have as some of these may shed light on the current diagnosis. About 85% of the time, a good and thorough history will lead to an accurate diagnosis even without the physical examination. The other 15% of the time, the cause of pain can be narrowed down to a list of possible diagnoses (called a differential diagnosis).

The examination will help to confirm the diagnosis suspected by the history and will narrow the possibilities that lead to the diagnosis. The spinal examination has to be performed meticulously so as not to miss subtle findings.

The diagnoses are reinforced with confirmatory tests. Imaging (x-rays, MRI, and others), electrical tests, and, occasionally, injections are involved.

A spine expert will also take the time to help you understand what the problem is, what the natural history is, and how treatment can help alleviate the problem. Most back problems need to be managed—not cured—and an understanding of the mechanics and physiology helps to alley concerns and get your life back in order again.

2

Terminology

Many common terms for lower back problems are infamously inaccurate. Descriptions date back sometime to the 1940s, a notorious time that is characterized by lack of spinal knowledge. Some of these ancient terms for some reason are still around today. To know the correct terms means you can have a better understanding and remove some of the stereotypes.

Lumbago simply means "low back pain." It does not describe any particular problem. If a doctor tells you your diagnosis is lumbago, you need another doctor.

A **strain** is simply an injury to a muscle or tendon. Strains are very common but are typically self-limiting (they heal quickly without treatment). A back strain should last one to twelve days. If it lasts longer, it may not be a strain.

A **sprain** is an injury to a ligament or a joint capsule. There are some ligaments in the spine that can be injured, but these are rarely a significant cause of pain. The sacroiliac joint is full of ligaments and can be injured, but this is also uncommon. Portions of the disc are made out of the same material as ligaments, but a disc tear is very different from a sprain. You could use the "sprain" term loosely for a disc tear, but it is poorly descriptive. A sprain is not a good term to use for the back.

The most common pain in the back is from an **annular tear**. This is the prototypical cause of acute lower back pain. Either the tear is preexisting and simply aggravated or a new tear has formed. This is normally what a "sprain" really is. This will be explained in great detail later in the book.

A **slipped disc** is not an accurate term. Discs can't slip as they are tightly attached to the vertebral bodies. Now, vertebral bodies can slip on each other, but this is a very different problem called a spondylolisthesis and will be discussed elsewhere in this book.

A **torn disc** is synonymous with a "degenerative disc" or an "annular tear" and not a good description of the problem.

A **bulging disc** is also a poor term. It can mean a weakness and an outpouching of the back wall of the disc or can mean an actual herniation. Again this is a nondescriptive term.

Sciatica is a term for nerve pain down the back of the leg from the sciatic nerve but is commonly used for any type of leg pain. Buttocks pain is normally sciatic pain.

A **herniated disc** means that the back wall of the disc is torn through and through, and a portion of the nucleus (the jelly) is protruding through.

An **extruded disc herniation** means that the jelly is now poking through the last structure to prevent it from actually touching the nerve, the PLL or posterior longitudinal ligament.

A **sequestered disc herniation** means that the jelly (nucleus) has pushed through the PLL and is a free fragment in the canal, no longer connected to the disc it came from.

Arthritis is a very poor term for the spine. This term is more appropriate for a peripheral joint such as a knee or hip where there is wearing of cartilage. The spine is programmed in many people to develop wear, and arthritis is not a good term for these individuals.

Degenerative disc disease is the term to define the entire degenerative cascade of the disc. It is a poor term by itself. It is popular (and I even use it) because the initials, **DDD**, are so easy to deal with. It is, however, not truly a disease, but a process due to genetics, injury, and occupation. Individuals with DDD may or may not have symptoms. It should be called DDS or degenerative disc syndrome, but I would spend all my time with my dentist trying to explain the difference between his back pain and his profession.

IDR or isolated disc resorption is an advanced form of DDD where the disc has fully reabsorbed, and the vertebrae are essentially sitting on top of each other, bone on bone. This situation creates its own set of peculiar symptoms but still may be asymptomatic in many individuals.

Scoliosis is a curvature of the spine in the coronal plane (looking at the individual from the front to back) greater than ten degrees. If it isn't ten degrees, it's not a scoliosis.

Kyphosis is the curve noted on the side view. The term, by itself, does not indicate pathology, but just describes the type of the curve. It is normal for thoracic spines to have kyphosis. An increased or decreased curve may note pathology.

Lordosis is the mirror-image curve to the kyphosis. It normally is found in the neck and lower back. Again, it is normal, and it does not indicate pathology unless increased or decreased beyond a certain point.

Cramping is a condition where the muscle goes into continuous spasm. Many times, leg cramping has nothing to do with the lumbar spine, but if there is a nerve compression, the muscle involved may more easily cramp. This needs to be differentiated from vascular and neurological disease that also causes cramping. Most cramping, however, is nothing to worry about.

Dystonia is an abnormal cramping of the muscle normally not caused by injury to the peripheral nervous system or muscle.

Peripheral neuropathy is a condition where the actual nerve itself is sick and sends abnormal signals to the brain (normally found in the legs).

Radiculopathy is inflammation of a single nerve root in the spinal canal normally from compression from a herniated disc.

3

The History of the Sources of Back and Leg Pain—"Pain Generators"

The biggest question for years regarding the lower back was where the pain originated. This issue had dogged physicians and therapists for years. Theories had abounded regarding why the spine hurts. Some blamed our two-legged stance for all our woes. Others implicated "bad posture." Our understanding of these "pain generators" has evolved in just over the last fifty years. It is interesting to look at some of the history and controversy regarding spine diagnosis and treatment. The old saw goes, "You can't know where you're going if you don't know where you've been."

Only since the development of Roentgen rays (x-rays) in 1895 have we developed a reasonable understanding of the disorders of the lower back. This new x-ray technique spread like wildfire. Literally within twelve months of its discovery, x-rays were being used for human diagnosis and not just in Germany but all over the world. X-rays were a substantial advance. Certainly, before this amazing invention, we knew what the spine and its supporting structures looked like anatomically through cadavers, but we really didn't know how aging and disorders manifested on the spinal column in a living subject. With x-rays, one could actually see the changes to the bone with the effects of aging or trauma in living subjects. Unfortunately, even with this advance, x-rays could visualize only bony structures. The nerves and discs of the spine continued to remain an obscurity at that time.

Disc problems were initially not understood. Why individuals repeatedly presented to doctors with severe leg pain and weakness was a mystery. An early physician, Dr. Walter Dandy of Johns Hopkins, theorized that there was something compressing the spinal nerves and, flouting conventional wisdom, surgically opened up the spinal canal in a patient. He found a mass in the canal compressing the nerves. Removal of this substance relieved the leg pain. Through Dr. Dandy, medical science finally found one of the first defining causes of leg pain. You would think this finding would be one of the "eureka" moments of medicine; however, this intracanal material was mistakenly thought to be a tumor instead of what its origin really was.

Dr. Mixter and Dr. Barr were the first to discover that this substance was actually material originating from the inside of the disc (what we now know as a herniated nucleus). This was a huge breakthrough. Only with this evidence did the understanding of degenerative spinal disorders take a great leap forward.

Finally, we had developed a reasonable understanding for some of the causes of leg pain. The sources of lower back pain, however, took many more years to be discovered. A very interesting study by Dr. Smith and Dr. Wright in back in the 1960s in England was one of the first to advance our knowledge. They performed back surgery to remove a herniated disc and, during surgery, tied multiple sutures to various anatomic structures. These tagged sutures were left long enough to protrude out of the incision after wound closure. When the patients awoke from anesthesia, the physicians would gently "tug" on these sutures and record the symptoms noted before the sutures were clipped off below the skin. Muscle, tendon, and ligament would generally not cause pain. Tension on the nerve would cause leg pain but not back pain, and tension on the back of the disc would cause back pain.

Dr. Kuslich from Minnesota expanded on this study. He performed surgery on patients with herniated discs with local anesthesia and sedation only. In other words, he did not put the patients to sleep but numbed the local structures similar to what a dentist does. The patients were awake enough to be able to describe sensations as the operation progressed.

Dr. Kuslich would first stimulate the skin and record the patient's reaction to this stimulus. He then would use a local numbing agent (similar to Novocain) to numb the skin, incise it, and dissect down to the fascia (the next structure immediately under the skin). Again, he would stimulate the fascia, record the patient's reaction, anesthetize this structure, incise it, and dissect down to the next structure.

He continued to dissect down layer by layer with stimulation. This brought him through the ligaments, muscle, bone, ligamentum flavum, capsule, and, finally, nerve and disc. His findings were extremely interesting.

Patients with low back pain almost never had significant reproduction of this pain when stimulating muscle or ligament. Only rarely would a facet joint cause typical low back pain. A "normal" (noncompressed or noninflammed) nerve never caused leg pain upon stimulation. It would only give a feeling of numbness or "pins and needles." An inflamed nerve (from a herniated disc) would cause exact reproduction of leg pain. Presuming the patient also had lower back pain, when the back of the disc (annulus) was stimulated, this would cause exact reproduction of their lower back pain. If the disc and nerve were stimulated at the same time, it would cause buttocks or sacroiliac pain.

Based upon these as well as many other studies, we now understand that most of the time, lower back pain originates from the disc. The facet joints, vertebral bodies, and spinal nerves can also be pain generators for lower back pain. Buttocks and leg pain primarily is generated from the nerve roots.

Now that we know where the sources of lower back and leg pain come from, we can use this information to make a more complete diagnosis. In addition, we can target each source to give much higher quality relief and solutions to pain in the spine and legs.

4

The Anatomy of the Lower Back (How It Looks and How It Works)

To understand anatomy for some can seem like "poking your eyes out." The subject is dry and can appear boring. Not understanding anatomy however is like trying to speak Spanish without knowing how to read it. When patients have disabling back pain, this topic does catch their attention, and they want to "learn the language."

The spine is really quite amazing in its construction. It has evolved over eons to the foundation that supports us today. We take our backbone for granted until we have pain and dysfunction.

The purpose of the spine seems self-evident but deserves repeating. The spine holds up the body. It allows enough motion to position the head and arms for the activities of daily living. The insult "You have a spine like a jellyfish" hits home here. The spine also protects the spinal cord from compression and injury. The spinal column through its discs and facets has to have shock-absorbing capability so impact doesn't injure the vertebrae and also has to be resistant to too much motion to prevent actions that would hurt the spinal cord and nerves.

Many people have made the argument that our unique ability to walk upright is the direct cause of our back problems. The truth is that many four-legged species develop significant back disorders after only three to six years. Humans normally don't develop problems until our thirties or forties. We have better spines than our dogs have. Upright posture however does create some unique problems that are not seen in quadrupeds. Our two-legged stance also creates research dilemmas as we don't have an animal model that walks only on two legs to study to help us study the mechanics of the spine.

Anatomy of the Lower Back

The lumbar spine is essentially a series of five building blocks called vertebrae. They stack up, one on top of the other. They sit on the sacrum, the triangular bone wedged into the pelvis. The sacrum is the "base bone" of the spine. The vertebrae are separated in front by the discs. The discs are the shock absorbers of the spine. They allow motion and yet absorb impact.

The back part of the spine contains the joints called the facets. These facets are the governors of spinal motion. They will allow bending forward, backward, and side to side but resist rotation. They also act as doorstops to prevent one vertebra from sliding forward on the one below.

The transverse processes stick out from the sides of the vertebrae and are essentially lever arms that muscles attach to. These levers allow smaller muscles to move the vertebral segments more easily. The spinous processes that project out the back of the vertebrae are also lever arms. Strong ligaments attach that prevent the spine from bending too far forward, and when bending backward, these processes abut, preventing too much backward motion. These spinous processes are the bumps seen on the back of anorexic models as they walk down the catwalk.

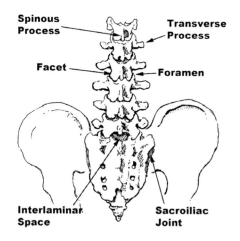

4-1A AP view of spine and pelvis

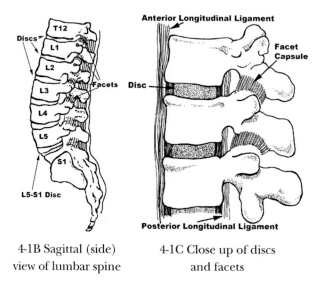

4-1B Sagittal (side)
view of lumbar spine

4-1C Close up of discs
and facets

Spinal Canal

The bony spinal canal sits in the center rear of the spine. It contains the spinal cord (which actually ends at the upper lumbar spine) and the nerves that exit out of the spinal cord (called the "cauda equina"—Latin for "horse's tail"). You can think of the spinal cord as an elongation of the brain. It is as sensitive to injury as the brain and has some functions similar to the lower end of the brain (the brain stem). The biggest difference is that the brain is housed in a rigid bony cavity for protection, and the spinal cord is housed in a moveable structure (the spinal column) that can and does wear out. This wear causes bone spurs and disc herniations that can compress the cord and therefore interfere with its function.

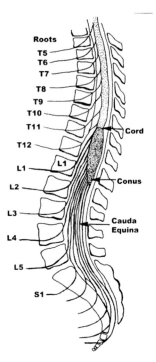

4-2 Spinal cord, conus and cauda equinal

An interesting fact is that the spinal cord at birth is long enough to reach the bottom of the spine; but as we grow, the vertebrae lengthen, but the spinal cord does not. Since the cord doesn't elongate, it is actually pulled up in the bony canal as the vertebrae enlarge and finally comes to rest in the upper lumbar spine. This is the reason why the spinal cord itself ends behind the body of L1. The nerves that attach to the lower cord compensate for this by stretching and lengthening (possibly one of the causes of "growing pains"). While the vertebrae lengthen, the spinal cord can become tethered, causing scoliosis and other symptoms (very rare).

The nerves in the lumbar spine below the end of the cord are all peripheral nerves, not central nerves. Peripheral nerves in general are much more resistant to compression and can heal if injured whereas the spinal cord generally doesn't. This fact comes into play if an injury is at a higher versus a lower level in the lower back.

As always, there is one exception. There is a small filamentous set of nerves called "nervi erigentes" in the cauda equina. These are the parasympathetic nerves that make the bowel and bladder function. These nerves come right out of the end of the spinal cord called the "conus medullaris." There is one rare emergent condition involving these nerves, usually caused by a large disc herniation called "cauda equina syndrome," generally a surgical emergency.

The spinal canal changes in diameter and volume with different positions. Bending forward enlarges the canal, making it 20% larger. Conversely, bending backward makes the canal 20% smaller. This change in volume has ramifications that will be discussed later in this book under spinal stenosis.

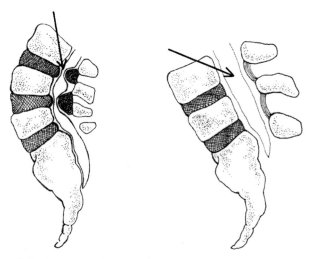

4-3 flexion extension canal diameter changes in stenosis

Facet Joints

In the back of the spine, the vertebrae are hooked together by paired joints called "facet joints." These facet joints are true joints similar to a hip or shoulder joint. A true joint (or diarthrodial joint) is essentially two bony surfaces covered with cartilage, a Teflon-type material, to reduce friction and allow the surfaces to glide with minimum resistance. The joint is surrounded by a capsule, effectively a stiff thick material that physically encloses and holds the joint together. The capsule prevents too much motion. The inside lining of this capsule are cells called the synovium that produce synovial fluid, the delicate fluid that lubricates the joint. There is a very thin layer of this within the joint itself, and the joint is actually under a vacuum. The pop that you feel when you crack your knuckles or a chiropractor manipulates your back is the breaking of this vacuum. It is not deleterious and sometimes can be beneficial.

These facet joints regulate directional motion as the discs by themselves don't have any directional stability. These joints allow you to bend forward and backward (flexion and extension), as well as bend side to side (lateral bending). The lower facet joints restrict rotation (twisting) more than the upper facets that, as you will see later, can cause some problems.

These facets also act as "doorstops." They hook from the vertebrae above onto the vertebrae below to prevent the superior vertebrae sliding forward on the lower one. This is important in the alignment of the lower two vertebrae. These two segments sit on a "ski slope" pointing downhill. The entire weight of the upper body rests on the two lower vertebrae, causing significant pressure to force them down this slope. The structures that resist this downward slide are the facets. They act as bony blocks (or doorstops) to prevent the slip. The discs by themselves offer little resistance to this forward force.

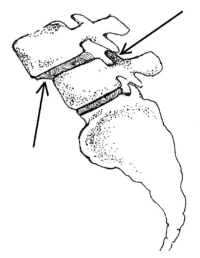

4-4 degenerative spondylolysthesis from facet
failure—arrows point to vertebral slip and facet wear

These facets can wear out and develop arthritis, just like any other joints. Bone spurs can form that press on the nearby nerves. There is a problematic condition where these doorstops break, called a spondylolisthesis. These pathological conditions will be discussed in another chapter.

Muscles of the Spine

The spine has muscles attached to induce and control motion. These muscles don't have the luxury to function like elbow or knee joint muscles do. A simple joint like the knee has muscles that cross in front and in back and directly attach to the bones on both sides of the joint. This gives them a simple task in contracting to manage the joint. In addition, the joints in the arms and legs are relatively intrinsically stable with ligaments and bony articulations that act as "stops." The spine is very different as it has many moveable segments, and there are no strong direct muscle attachments for three of the six directions it can bend.

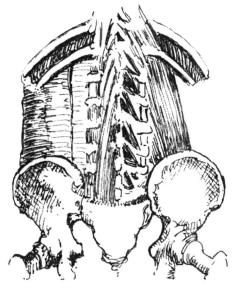

4-5 multifidi and transversalis muscle

Since the spine can bend forward, backward, bend in the right and left lateral directions, and rotate both left and right, the muscles that control the spine have significantly more work and coordination to do than any other region in the body. The muscles that *directly* attach from one vertebra to another are unfortunately short and weak. The major muscles that have the strength to control spinal movements and position bypass the individual vertebra and connect indirectly to the spine through other structures. These are called the core muscles.

The Core Muscles

What are the muscles that make up the core? To understand the muscles is to understand the bony structures that the muscles attach to. The ribs attach to the midback (thoracic spine) and surround the chest extending to the front where they join at the sternum. These ribs create one of the fulcrum points for the core muscles in front and in back. The pelvis is the other structure that these muscles attach to.

Muscles in the front (rectus abdominis, transversalis, external and internal obliques) attach from the ribs to the front and sides of the pelvis. These muscles don't attach directly to the spine, but they will create spinal rigidity by increasing abdominal pressure and indirectly stiffening the spine. These muscles can be strengthened to also prevent or assist rotation of the pelvis and stabilize extension (backward bending).

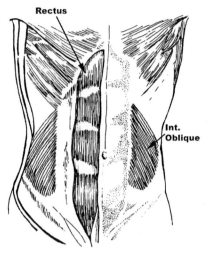

4-6 Anterior core muscles

The lumbar extensors or muscles in the back (quadratus lumborum and erector spinae) attach from the sacrum and pelvis to the thoracic spine. There are some small attachments to the lumbar spine, but the attachments generally start at the vertebra and *ascend* not descend. There are no muscles in the rear of the spine that go from the pelvis directly to the vertebra except for the some branches of the quadratus lumborum! This entire grouping of muscles is the primary control to resist flexion (bending forward) and direct lateral bending.

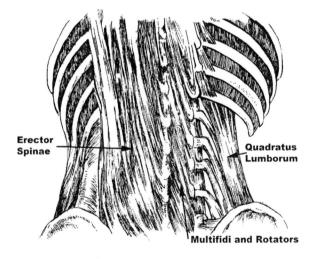

4-7 posterior core muscles

The intrinsic muscles are the very small muscles that connect directly from one vertebra to another. These are the multifidi, intertransversarii, and interspinales. These are quite diminutive muscles and can't generate a significant amount of force. Nonetheless, they can be helpful as important stabilizers of individual vertebra.

Pelvic Muscular Control

The pelvis is often forgotten as a control mechanism of the lower back. The pelvis can act in two ways. First, it is considered the "base bone of the spine" as the sacrum is the foundation of the spinal column. If the pelvis is tilted forward (called anterior rotation), this causes an increased lumbar lordosis. Conversely, if tilted backward (posterior rotation), this flattens the lumbar spine or reduces the lordosis.

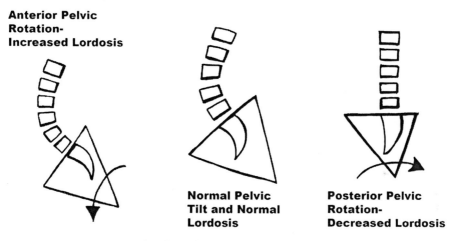

Anterior Pelvic Rotation- Increased Lordosis

Normal Pelvic Tilt and Normal Lordosis

Posterior Pelvic Rotation- Decreased Lordosis

4-8 Pelvic tilt and effect on lordosis

The other function of the pelvis is as an intercalated segment. The pelvis will move with the lumbar spine by rotating at the hip joint to act as a shock absorber that reduces stress on the spine.

The pelvis has two swivel points, one at the hip attachment and one at the spine attachment. Muscles insert at approximately four points on the pelvis and can tip or rotate it depending on the amount of muscular contraction.

Tight hamstrings will pull the pelvis down in back (causing posterior rotation) that levels the sacral base and reduces lordosis. Some patients with a slip of L5 (spondylolisthesis) will unconsciously contract the hamstrings to reduce the slope of the vertebra to prevent further slip and stress on the structures.

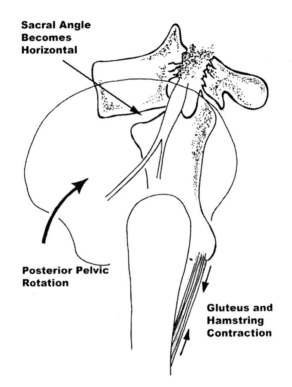

Sacral Angle Becomes Horizontal

Posterior Pelvic Rotation

Gluteus and Hamstring Contraction

4-9 Tight hamstrings and reduction of slip angle of L5

5

Physiology Of The Disc (What Can Go Wrong)

Mechanically, everything in the lumbar spine revolves around the disc. The disc functions like a shock absorber. This structure absorbs impact and still allows for motion of the spine. It also has to have restraints to prevent damage to itself and the other spinal structures such as the nerves and facets. These requirements create some major demands.

The disc originates from the notochord, the very primitive first structure seen when the fetus is just beginning to form as an embryo. Even when adults, there still are cells of this primitive notochord that can be found within the disc. A very rare form of cancer generated from only these cells can form in the spine.

In appearance, the disc looks like a jelly donut. The jelly (called the nucleus) is made of sugars attached to a protein backbone called a proteoglycan. This structure allows it to act like a giant sponge. The jelly pulls in water from the body of the vertebra to create a high-pressure interior matrix (think of the jelly as the air pressure in a tire).

The outside of the donut is made up of about thirty rings of collagen called the annulus, just like the plies of a tire. These rings are normally quite tough. Each layer of these rings alternates in angulation in their attachment to the bone of the vertebra.

The end plates of the disc separate the bone of the vertebral body from the interior of the disc. They are made of hyaline cartilage—the same cartilage that lines the hip and knee joints. This material creates a barrier to nutrients and oxygen entering and exiting the disc.

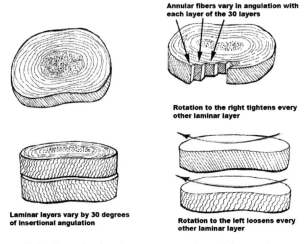

5-1A Annular laminar construction with rotation
reducing load on half of annular fibers

Blood Supply and Imbibition

Problems exist with the design of the disc that causes the "disease" we know today as degenerative disc disease or DDD. The first problem is that the blood supply, for all intensive purposes, disappears from the disc by about the age of eight (yes, eight). This means that collectively, the discs are the largest structures in the body that have no blood supply.

Without a blood supply, there is very poor oxygen penetration into the interior of the disc. The only fluids that can be exchanged are under hydrostatic and osmotic pressure. This means that motion of the disc exchanges fluids similarly to a squeezing a sponge underwater and releasing it. The water and nutrients that this material absorbs and releases transfers through the end plate of the vertebra under a process called imbibition.

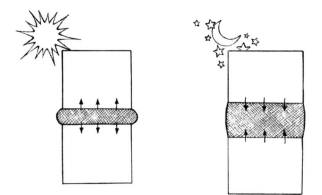

5-2 Height change of disc with day and night

This effect is evident with prolonged standing. When individuals stand up in the morning, they have more water pressure in the disc and are actually about one-fourth-to one-half-inch taller than they are in the evening. The pressure inside the disc with prolonged standing forces water out, making the discs thinner, and therefore, people are shorter in the evening. When lying down to sleep, the pressure drops, and fluid absorbs again inside the disc, repeating the process. It is interesting to note that astronauts seem to get more advanced degenerative disc disease the longer they spend time in space. It seems that lack of load on the disc may lead to reduced transfer of nutrients and accelerated degenerative changes.

The fluids that are transferred into the disc are poor in oxygen and limited in nutrients. This creates a problem for the living cells inside the disc. These cells produce the glycoproteins that make up the nucleus (the gel or sponge), and they need oxygen to function well. Without oxygen, these cells become much less effective keeping up with maintaining the jelly. This lack of oxygen is called an anaerobic environment. Without the production and maintenance of these gel proteins, the pressure in the disc drops with age. Interestingly, take these cells out of the disc and put them in a culture medium with normal amounts of oxygen and they function normally, indicating that blood supply and nutritional lack is the problem, not the cells becoming "old."

Pressure Drop

When the pressure drops inside the disc, this is similar to letting some air out of a car tire. As the pressure in the car tire drops, the sidewalls bulge outward from the weight of the car. When you then try to drive on a partially filled tire, there is less stability to hold the road, especially with unpredicted maneuvers such as a quick turn to avoid an obstacle or driving over an unexpected speed bump. Just as the car has trouble holding the road, a degenerative disc is much less resistant to abnormal movements, and these motions can tear the disc wall. An injury or unexpected lift or fall may injure the disc.

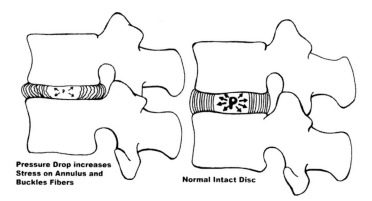

**Pressure Drop increases
Stress on Annulus and
Buckles Fibers**

Normal Intact Disc

5-3 Pressure drop of nucleus causes increased stress on disc wall

Annular Tears and Nociceptors

If a tear occurs, without a blood supply, the disc can't heal if injured. All injuries to the disc therefore are cumulative or add up. To say it another way, any injury to the disc is essentially a permanent injury. A tear of the collagen in the donut won't repair itself. The cells lining the outside wall of the annulus attempt to repair the outer defect but are unsuccessful and actually get in the way.

There is a tenuous blood supply in the outer one-third of the disc. Tears that go out to here will attempt to heal, but the scar tissue laid down is not nearly as strong as the collagen fibers it attempts to replace. To make matters worse, any blood vessels that grow into the torn fibers of the disc carry along with them new pain fibers. These fibers are highly sensitive and another major cause of pain sensitization of the disc.

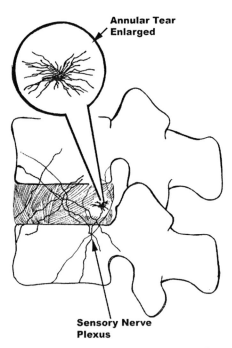

Annular Tear Enlarged

Sensory Nerve Plexus

5-4 Tear of annulus causes ingrowth
of vessels and pain nerves

There have been some bizarre discoveries regarding the chemical nature of the nucleus (jelly). The nucleus or interior of the disc has been demonstrated to contain many compounds that are, by themselves, direct causes of inflammation. That is, these chemicals taken out of the disc and placed anywhere in the body will cause a nerve to become sick. Arachidonic acid, metaloproteases, and substance P are only some of these noxious substances. Why these molecules are part of the inside of the disc that resides immediately next to the nerve roots is one of life's great mysteries.

The back portion of the disc (posterior annulus) is full of pain sensors called nociceptors. When a tear occurs in the annulus of the disc, these pain receptors come in contact with the nucleus of the disc. The pain receptors themselves then become inflamed and much more easily transmit pain signals.

Your Mom and Dad

The second problem with the disc is how you picked your mom and dad—genetics. This has to do with the type of collagen that makes up the plies of the tire (the annulus). The collagen in the annulus is not uniform. Some fibers are pliable and resilient and can undergo multiple loading cycles without any wear just like thick bungee cords. Other types of collagen are unfortunately brittle, like wire coat hangers. You can bend these only a limited amount of times before they break from fatigue failure.

Good examples of this genetic relationship are the variety of patients I am asked to see. Some are injured on the ski slopes. Eighty—and, occasionally, ninety-year-olds (and yes, they ski in Vail) will sporadically develop pain in their backs and have an MRI performed through the emergency room. There are times these octo—and nonagenarians have perfect-looking discs (they obviously picked the right parents). On the other end of the spectrum are the unfortunate twelve-year-olds in my practice with severe degenerative disc disease.

Remember Wiring!

There is a big caveat here. Remember, just because the patient may have degenerative disc disease does not mean they are going to have symptoms of low back pain. A study out of Emery University noted that more than 60% of individuals without back or leg pain had degenerative changes in their discs. These people *had no symptoms.* I am always reminded of this when I see older NFL players with horrible-looking spines and minimal to no pain. This leads into the theory of wiring.

There are two groups of patients with the same problems found on x-rays and MRI. One group has no symptoms, and the other may be incapacitated with the same type of degenerative spine. It appears that some individuals are "wired" to have low back pain, and others are not. This effect has to do with the sensitivity of the central nervous system and the number of pain receptors present and active in the area of injury. For example, I personally have a degenerative disc at L5-S1 and have virtually no low back pain. Others with the same type of disc on MRI are incapacitated. I have lousy wiring and am so grateful that my spine is so uneducated.

6

Nerve Anatomy and Physiology

In order to understand pain and why it occurs, you need to understand the nervous system and how it works. The nervous system is divided into three parts: the central nervous system, the peripheral nervous system, and the autonomic nervous system. The central nervous system (CNS) consists of the brain and spinal cord. This is where consciousness or "the sense of self" occurs. The peripheral nervous system (PNS) consists of all the sensors and nerves that relay outside information to the CNS and conveys messages from the brain to the body. The autonomic nervous system (ANS) is the "housekeeping system" and has two components: the sympathetic and parasympathetic systems that oppose each other.

Autonomic Nervous System

The autonomic system (sympathetic and parasympathetic) keeps track of the bodily functions without needing conscious attention—hence the term "autonomic" (automatic). The sympathetic portion of this system can be thought of as responsible for the "fight or flight" reaction. When this system gets stimulated, the heart races, the adrenal glands pump epinephrine into the blood, the skeletal muscles become engorged, the sweat glands activate, and all the body systems are "ready for action." This is a very ancient arrangement that was very important for survival of the human race.

In the old days, when a dinosaur was after a human (or maybe nowadays a mugger), this revving up gives the human body the ability to perform at a much greater speed and capacity. Even though this system has been studied thoroughly, there are still substantial unknowns. The general thought at one time was that this system is a one-way pathway going strictly from our lower brain centers to the body, not from the body to the brain. There is now some evidence that this system has a "sensory" component that registers as deep pain separate from the normal nervous system. Reflex sympathetic dystrophy, a chronic pain condition, is an example.

The other component of this autonomic system is the parasympathetic constituent. This is the "housekeeping" part of the system that is important in digestion, reproduction, and elimination. It slows down the heart, helps to secrete enzymes for digestion, and controls the function of the sexual organs. This system is also important for bowel and bladder function. When someone "faints," their parasympathetic system has become overstimulated so that the heart rate slows down considerably, and insufficient blood gets pumped to the head, causing a temporary loss of consciousness. This is called a vasovagal event.

Spinal Autonomic Nervous System

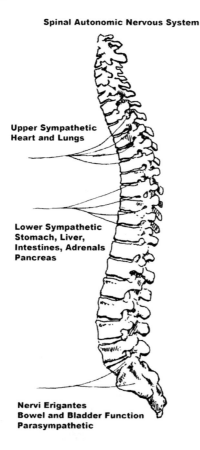

**Upper Sympathetic
Heart and Lungs**

**Lower Sympathetic
Stomach, Liver,
Intestines, Adrenals
Pancreas**

**Nervi Erigantes
Bowel and Bladder Function
Parasympathetic**

6-1 Autonomic nervous system in the spine

Anatomy of a Nerve Cell

The nerve cell is the longest single cell in the body, with some reaching up to three feet in length. There are two ends: the axon and the dendrite. The *cell body* of the nerve is its "brain" and storehouse and is situated between the two ends. If the cell body dies, so does the nerve. However, if the nerve is part of the peripheral system (PNS) and the end of the nerve dies distant from the cell body, under certain conditions, the nerve can regenerate.

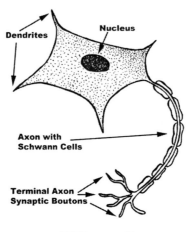

6-2 Nerve cell

Nerves need to be stimulated to fire. They are like the wiring in a home. The triggering stimulus depends upon the sensor attached to the end of the nerve similar to a smoke alarm or doorbell. A smoke alarm won't respond to finger pressure, and a doorbell won't respond to smoke. When the sensor triggers the nerve, the nerve sends an electrical signal down to the other end to deliver the message. There are some nerves that have raw endings (no sensors) and will trigger with local cell damage.

The nerves don't actually touch at the ends. When the signal finally gets to the end of the nerve through the axon, it has to cross a gap to the next nerve. This gap is called the synapse. The nerve communicates with the next nerve using a chemical signal called a neurotransmitter. When the nerve is simulated and fired, the message is sent down the nerve to the end, and then it releases this chemical neurotransmitter by spraying the next nerve through this synapse.

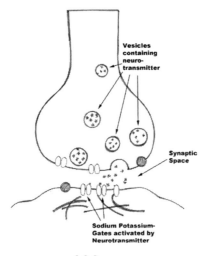

6-3 Synapse

For the peripheral nerves, the neurotransmitter is typically a substance called acetylcholine. This means that when the brain sends a signal down to contract a muscle, the end of this nerve releases this chemical by spraying across this gap. The next nerve continues the signal, or if the nerve is connected to a muscle, the muscle responds to this sprayed chemical by contracting.

If the nerve itself is compressed or inflamed, it may not be able to conduct the message, so the sensor connected to the nerve will be muted (numbness) or release acetylcholine, and the muscle can't contract (weakness). In a disease process called myasthenia gravis, the acetylcholine in the end of the nerve is inactivated, and the nerve can't release enough to contract the muscles. The patient becomes very weak.

Myelination or Not?

Some nerves are myelinated. This means that they have a fatty coating surrounding them called a myelin sheath. There are regular breaks in this coating (the nodes of Ranvier). The electrical signal that travels down the nerve literally jumps from node to node (a process called saltitory conduction). The speed of this conduction is ten to twenty times greater than unmyelinated nerves, so the signal gets to and from the brain faster than a simple nerve without myelin. There is a disease process called multiple sclerosis that attacks the myelin sheath, so the conduction slows down or stops, and patients can lose control of their muscles and have abnormal sensations.

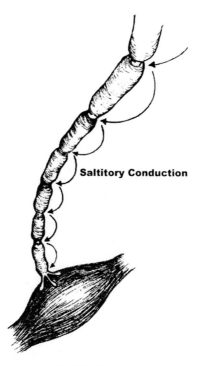

Saltitory Conduction

6-4 Myelination

The myelin can also be injured by compression such as a herniated disc. The myelin cells can repair themselves, but it may take four to twelve weeks for recovery.

Nerves are categorized as to size and whether they are myelinated or unmyelinated. There are four groups of nerves: alpha, beta, gamma, and delta. Alpha fibers concern motor, proprioception (sense of position), and reflex (the hammer on the knee a doctor uses). Beta fibers are associated with muscle innervation (contraction), touch, and pressure. Gamma fibers hook to muscle spindles (to tell your brain what the muscles are doing), and delta fibers are involved with pain and temperature. There are also B fibers that are thinly myelinated preganglionic autonomic axons (huh?) that innervate smooth muscle (intestines). C fibers are unmyelinated and are conduits for nociceptor (pain) impulses.

The Stimulus

A stimulus is needed to cause the receptor attached to the nerve to fire to send a signal. The stimulus needs to be strong enough and of the right type to "get the nerve's attention." The smallest amount of stimulation needed to trigger a nerve is called the threshold stimulus. Stimulation below this threshold will not trigger the nerve. Nerves can be inflamed (made more sensitive) so that a much smaller stimulation will trigger the nerve. This happens when certain chemicals come in contact with the nerve (think of the back of the disc and the noxious jelly) or the nerve itself is injured.

If the nerve is constantly stimulated, this causes the nerve to become more sensitive, and it will trigger more easily. This process is called facilitation. Pain that moves up a nerve pathway will have an easier time moving up that pathway the second time and even easier the third time. You now can see how chronic pain can "reproduce itself" and become an unwanted permanent part of the nervous system. Interestingly enough, this is also, grossly, how learning and memory in the brain works.

Sensors

The way the human body gets information from the outside world is through sensors at the beginnings of the peripheral (and cranial) nerves. Sensors, like rods and cones in the eyes, are responsive to light. In low light levels, the eye can only see in black-and-white images as the rods are more responsive to low light than color receptors (cones). Small hairlike cells in the ear are responsive to vibration (hearing), and taste buds in the mouth are obviously sensitive to chemicals (taste).

Sensory nerves give feedback regarding the environment. Light touch on the skin causes sensors (Meissner's Corpuscles) to trigger the nerve to fire. This information is carried to the brain through a number of pathways where it arrives in the cerebral cortex, and the individual experiences the sensation of touch. Similar sensations occur with temperature, deep touch, and vibration through different nerve pathways.

Interestingly enough, with the same stimulus, the limbic part of the brain may interpret this sense of touch as either pleasurable or disgusting, depending upon the context of the situation.

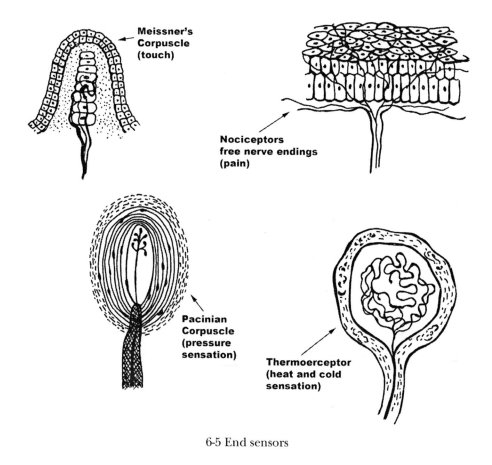

6-5 End sensors

Proprioception

There are multiple sensor cells in the arms, legs, and trunk that specialize in different types of input. Stretch receptors are located in the muscles, tendons, and joints (called muscle spindles, golgi tendon organs, and capsular receptors, respectively). They respond to the tension in the muscles, tendons, and joints regarding the position of the body. This is why one can close their eyes and still sense where body parts are in space. The input from these sensors arrives in the brain, and there is a subconscious "image" of where the body is. This sensation is called proprioception, and there are more peripheral nerves dedicated to this sense than any other.

Balance

Balance is a complicated feedback mechanism that uses this proprioception sense and automatic muscle contraction. Balance is mainly regulated by the lower part of the brain, the cerebellum. Information is conveyed through the proprioception system to the cerebellum, the rear portion of the brain. The vestibular mechanism in the ear also contributes to the cerebellum. It acts like a gyroscope so the brain knows up from down. These systems through the cerebellum give unconscious messages to the muscles of the trunk and legs to keep the body upright and balanced. There is a condition called cervical myelopathy—narrowing of the spinal canal in the neck—that causes interruption of signals at the spinal cord level and creates imbalance and incoordination of hands and legs.

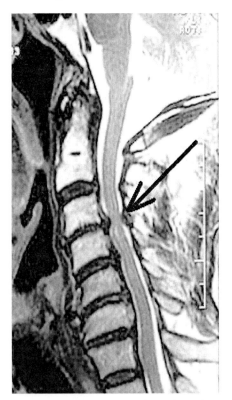

6-6 Cervical stenosis and myelopathy

The Reflex Arc

The reflexes in the muscles and tendons are an important part of this balance mechanism and are one of the simplest nerve reflex loops we have. When you stand and imperceptibly start to lean forward, the muscles and tendons in the back of your leg will slightly stretch. This triggers the stretch receptors in these structures to fire, and an automatic correction will occur by contraction of these same muscles. The muscle contraction resists the forward lean and returns you to a neutral balanced position. These corrections occur hundreds of times a second and are relatively unconscious.

This is the part of the reflex arc that your doctor checks with his reflex hammer. A tap to the knee stretches the patellar tendon. Through this reflex arc, the nerve transfers the message to the spinal cord, the corresponding motor nerve fires, the quadriceps muscle contracts, and your knee jerks. The sensory nerve connected to the tendon stretch receptor, the spinal cord, the motor nerve, and the muscle are tested by this reflex. A problem with any one of these structures will dull or even excite this reflex. It is an unconscious reflex, but you can consciously resist it by tightening the muscles around the knee. These reflexes tend to dull with advancing age.

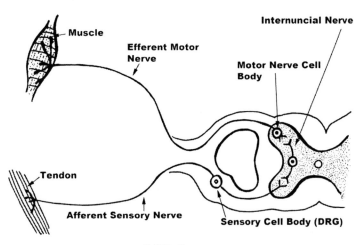

6-7 Reflex arc

Nerve Root

The nerve root is a special part of the structure of the peripheral nerve. It is the area of the nerve that is between the end of the spinal cord and the dorsal root ganglia (DRG). The DRG is located right at the exit where the nerve exits the spinal canal. After the DRG, the nerve becomes a peripheral nerve and has structure that makes it tougher and more resistant to stretch and compression.

The nerve root in the spinal canal is made up of pain nerves, sensory nerves (position sense, sharp and light touch, and temperature), and motor nerves. The dorsal root ganglion is the home of the sensory nerve cell bodies. These bodies are more sensitive to injury than the normal axon of the nerve. Compression of this root will cause paresthesias (pins and needles sensation), decreased sensation, and possibly weakness of muscles in the distribution of this root. We have mapped these roots, and therefore, we can develop a diagnosis of which nerve root is involved based on symptoms and physical examination.

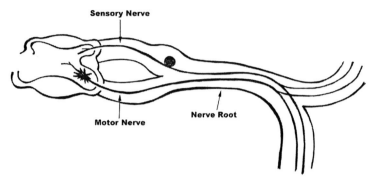

6-8 Nerve root and dorsal root ganglia

7

Pain

Just like proprioception or touch, pain is simply another piece of sensory information regarding our environment. Special nerve endings permeate our body. Some of these are "raw" nerve endings. They have no receptors attached to them. Others have sensors called nociceptors attached to their end. These are specifically designed to register tissue injury by chemical, pressure, or temperature receptors. All of these sensors give us protective information regarding damage to our tissues so we can react accordingly, i.e., "Remove your hand from the hot stove, stupid."

So why do we need these pain nerves, and would we be better off without them? There are two examples to help you understand the need for pain input. Both regard the absence of these sensors.

The first example is the genetic disorder called *congenital insensitivity to pain.* These individuals were born without pain feedback to their brain. They commonly lose their fingers and toes through burns and injuries because they are insensitive to the tissue injury. Cigarette smokers will burn their fingertips because they can't feel heat. Some lose toes because they can't feel the pressure of constricting shoes or socks.

The second example is patients with spinal cord injuries. Without feedback from their sensory system, they develop abnormal motion of the spine. Many develop severely destroyed joints (called Charcot joints after the famous French physician) that become very dysfunctional and painful.

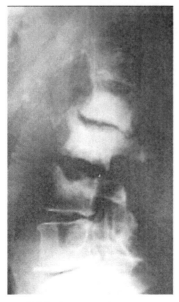 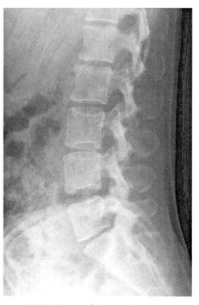

7-1A charcot spine—note   7-1B Normal lateral x-ray
sclerosis and destruction
of motion segments

This joint destruction could not occur without loss of the protective pain and sensory nerves. This does beg the question as why they have pain even though they are suppose to have no sensation. They have lost the connection from their brain to their body, but we theorize that sympathetic nerves of the autonomic nervous system (not associated with the spinal nerves) carry a deep pain signal that these patients feel.

Genetic Perception of Pain (Why We Are So Low-Back Ignorant)

Our brains have evolved in a way that predetermines our sensory input or how much we can consciously pay attention to any one area of the body. In other words, our sensory cortex is wired to "pay more attention" to certain areas of the body at the expense of other areas. The wonderful diagram from Dr. Frank Netter demonstrates how our sensory input is preprogrammed genetically.

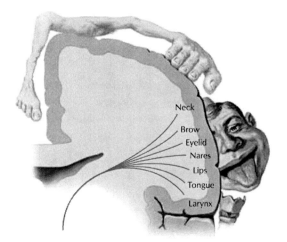

7-2 Homonculus—This diagram indicates how much
of the surface area of the brain is devoted to
sensation of the respective parts of the body
Copyright by Elsevier

The index fingertip has thousands of pain and sensory fibers and just as many "receiver cells" at the cerebral cortex, where we can note the sensation consciously. A paper cut can be perceived by the sensory cortex at its exact location on the fingertip. Even with the eyes closed, it is easy to recognize the location of any injury on the hand, tongue, face, or any surface that is imbued with multitudes of sensory end organs.

Regarding the spine, especially the lumbar spine, you can see from the diagram that there is a very poor allocation of pain and sensory fibers to the sensory cortex. No one has ever come into my office stating, "Doc, I can tell, it's my L4-5 disc on the right, I think I tore part of my annulus." We are so poorly allocated in the sensory cortex of our brains as to location of lumbar injuries that we can only recognize back pain but not what area or what structure. Most back pain is described as deep, dull, nonspecific pain. That is because of our "hard wiring." We really don't have the sensors to identify exactly where the pain is coming from.

Referral Pain

Not all buttocks, hip, and leg pain originates from the nerve root or from the hip joint. There is a common phenomenon called referred pain. This is pain that does not derive from the actual area that "feels" painful, but from a distant site. This pain isn't a direct result of a nerve radiating pain down the leg. We know from research and by experience that it is generated by an injured part *not in connection* with the painful area. There is no thorough knowledge of why or how this pain occurs. The symptoms are thought to occur by crossover stimulation of pain fibers up in the spinal cord or by the sympathetic system. In embryology, the pain generating and receiving parts are related by a region called the sclerotome. It then makes sense to call it sclerotomal pain.

We have however mapped these pain generators. In some simple experiments, Bogduk, Dwyer, and Cloward have irritated structures in a conscious (awake) patient, and the patient has then reported their symptoms. The structures (discs and facets) were irritated with a saline solution using simple pressure. The patient noted symptom pattern pain that radiated to areas not directly connected to the structures.

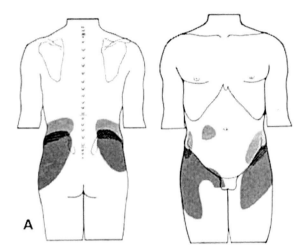

7-3 Referral pain pattern from injections into the facets (Bogduk)

A good example of this referral pain is the discomfort commonly felt in the poor maligned sacroiliac joint. Many patients and even some therapists blame the sacroiliac joint itself for much of the pain that commonly occurs here. It makes logical sense since the SI joint is at the center of the pain, and when pressing on the joint, it can be very tender. The SI joint, however, only very rarely causes pain. Almost all of sacroiliac pain originates from the lower lumbar discs and nerves. This can be proven by numbing the lower lumbar discs and nerves and watching the SI pain disappear.

Another example of referral pain is a set of symptoms commonly called piriformis syndrome. The piriformis is a small muscle in the back of the hip area that lies right next to and occasionally on the sciatic nerve. There are times that the sciatic nerve can go right through the muscle, splitting it. Early anatomists noted this and, since the cause of sciatica was not understood at the time, deduced that this muscle should be the cause of painful sciatica. Since the sciatic nerve generates pain, the pain commonly refers to this muscle. The muscle becomes very tender, and early anatomists can't be blamed for indicting this muscle as the origin of the pain. With exceptions, the piriformis is an innocent bystander and, normally, not the cause of sciatica.

Pain Filters

We are all wired differently (neurologically). This means that two individuals with the same injury will have different pain intensities and locations. The same pain stimulus at different times in the same person can be experienced differently also. The response to the pain is not just based how the nervous system is hardwired to handle the pain, but also on personality or past experience and the physiological situation at the time. The memory also plays a role in pain handling. Anticipation of pain causes anxiety that in turn amplifies pain.

This occurs in two different ways. The first is the general reaction to pain. Simplifying things, we have a pain filter between our conscious brain and our body. Some of us have very dense filters and feel very little pain. A case in point is an individual that enters the emergency room with an amputated finger. It's amazing, but many are in no discomfort whatsoever. The next individual who shows up in the ER may have a small finger laceration but needs large amounts of narcotics just to tolerate this injury. This individual has more porous pain filters.

Social situations can affect these pain filters subconsciously. A person who was injured on the job or who was hurt in a motor vehicle accident feels that his or her life is altered but not by his or her own fault. Sometimes these individuals lose their desire and responsibility for getting better because "someone else did this to me." When there is blame involved, subconsciously, this filter can become more porous, and the pain becomes harder to control.

This does not rule out a significant injury to spinal structures and the pain not being real, but means that treating this injury can be more difficult unless the pain filter can be made more functional or the pain process can be remedied. Depression and anxiety also amplify pain.

Hard Wiring and Bone Pain

This difference can also be noted in how some of our structures are hardwired. The disc is a good example. Some patients have severe degenerative disc disease with many tears in the back of the disc. Because they may have very few or insensitive pain receptors, they feel minimal or no pain. Others can have a small posterior tear with a relatively normal disc on MRI and have severe incapacitating low back pain.

Bone wiring also appears to be very different. The disc, as noted previously, acts as a shock absorber. Impact activities such as running, tennis, skiing, and basketball cause shock to the spine. The disc is designed to absorb this shock and dissipate it. When the disc becomes incompetent, this shock is transferred to the bone in the body of the vertebra, which is a rigid structure. The shock can cause damage to this bone in the form of stress fracturing. The symptoms are normally a deep, dull ache, but this can occur hours after the activity. As a case in point, I have a very degenerative disc in the lower back; with these changes, I have no lower back pain. I am simply not hardwired to feel this pain.

Abnormal Pain Transmission (Neuropathic Pain)

There are times however, on the other end of the spectrum, that the nerves send pain signals even though there is no damaged bone or tissue. This occurs when the nerve itself become injured. It is somewhat like a short circuit. When this happens, the nerves can trigger much more easily or even spontaneously without stimulation. They send pain signals even though there is no tissue damage to trigger them. This type of pain is called *neuropathic pain*. It can lead to a syndrome called *chronic pain syndrome*. Phantom pain syndrome is a well-known example. This phenomenon is where individuals who have had an amputation of a limb still have pain in the limb. A patient with a below-the-knee amputation will have pain in their foot. The pain is generated by the injured nerves that are severed from the amputation, but the other ends still connect to the spinal cord.

Conclusion

So pain is an important sensation for survival. It is designed for self-preservation or to prevent injury. As you can see, pain can be caused by tissue injury but can also be a false signal by an actual injury to the nerve itself. Also, if the nerve is sensitized, regardless if it is injured or not, pain messages will be transmitted more easily (remember facilitation?), and smaller stimuli that would not trigger the nerve normally may trigger the nerve now.

8

Typical Disorders That Cause Back and Leg Pain

This is an important chapter to recognize what can go wrong with the spine. By understanding the previous chapters, you can now speculate that the spine is ripe for problems. This chapter is dedicated to the typical everyday mechanical disorders of the spine that cause 95% of all back and leg pain. Disorders can be divided into problems that cause only back pain, problems that cause only leg pain, combination back and leg problems, and, finally, problems of spinal alignment. All of these disorders are interrelated. That is, a patient may have back pain from a degenerative disc and an eventual collapse of that disc on one side that compresses the nerve causing leg pain.

Causes of Back Pain

Acute Annular Tear

"My back went out." This is the most common refrain for the most frequent acute disorder of the spine. These tears occur in the back of the annulus, the plies of the tire that holds the nucleus (the jelly) inside. They can occur with simple or complex activity. Normally the onset of the annular tear is with a twist or bend of the lower back and the sensation of a slight "give" or "pop." Tears are quite common and many times are not painful. The reason some individuals are incapacitated with pain and others have no symptoms is a Nobel Prize-winning answer.

Onset of pain may be immediate but typically may be delayed a half hour to a day after the incident. The patient will be sore and stiff with pain inhibition of the core muscles. This will cause a "locking up" of the muscles, and getting out of bed may be an ordeal. The spine will feel tight and "out of sorts." The manifestation of these symptoms may simply fade away or may continue to increase and become more painful. If the injury is a simple tear, the symptoms will disappear within two days to three weeks and generally will cause no further problems.

The cause of pain is an inflammation of the pain nerves in the torn fibers in the annulus. The feedback mechanism that causes these symptoms has yet to be fully elucidated but nonetheless shuts down the muscles of the back, making any movements seem like dragging a thousand-pound weight around by the waist.

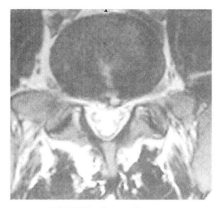

8-1 MRI of annular tear

Degenerative Disc Disease

This is the most common cause of chronic lower back pain. The age of occurrence is normally older than thirty with a peak in the late thirties and early forties. There is a subset of patients with a genetic predisposition that can occur as early as the teens. Degenerative disc disease is a cascade of events with the first step being a drop in the pressure in the center (nucleus) of the disc. The disc loses stiffness, and the annulus (the plies of the tire) bares more stress than it is designed to tolerate. The annulus then suffers multiple episodes of tears (see annular tears above). The nerve fibers in the tears become chronically inflamed by exposure to the nucleus. Similar to a bad shock absorber on a car, the disc develops microinstability.

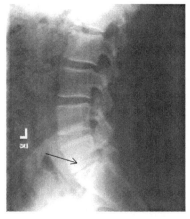

8-2 X-ray lateral of isolated disc resorption—
arrow points to degenerated disc

The location of symptoms is the center of the low back, but the pain can occasionally radiate to the groin, sacroiliac joint, or buttocks (referral pain). The quality of pain is typically dull and will increase with prolonged loading. Sharp pain can develop with instability maneuvers (sneezing, bending, lifting, or stepping off an unexpected curb). The back pain will typically be worse toward the end of the day, but the patient can also exhibit morning stiffness and pain. When the pain radiates into the groin, it mimics hip disorders.

These symptoms can be confused with deconditioned muscle pain that occurs with activities that been done infrequently such as spring gardening or a long run. Deconditioned muscle pain goes away with time and doesn't normally recur. Disc pain is consistently repeated with the same activities.

Does occupation or lifestyle have any bearing on the chances of a greater propensity to develop degenerative disc disease? Interestingly, there are very few current indications that occupation will change the chance of developing DDD. One particular study however noted that truck and bus drivers had a higher incidence of disc problems. Vibration of the vehicles they drove was absorbed into the lumbar spine.

The lumbar spine has the same resonance as the vibration of a truck or bus and absorbs this energy. The reason is that objects have a natural frequency at which they vibrate. Take a guitar or violin and put it in front of a speaker. If a C note is played over the speaker, only the C string will vibrate on the instrument as it absorbs this energy. The other strings won't vibrate because they don't resonate at the same frequency. If you look at a bus driver's seat, you may notice that it has an air ride component (it floats on a cushion of air) to isolate the driver from the vibration of the vehicle.

You might assume that a ditchdigger, roofer, or heavy mechanic would have a greater chance of degenerative spine changes, but there are no current studies that support this conclusion.

Isolated Disc Resorption (IDR)

This condition is considered the tail end of the degenerative disc disease cascade. Most discs rarely get to this point. With isolated disc resorption, the disc has fully degenerated and essentially either turns into an old piece of shoe leather or just wears away completely. There is no cushion left between the vertebral bodies where there is bone-on-bone contact. The vertebral bodies take the brunt of any impact. There may be some microinstability (abnormal motion of the old disc space), but the main problem is structural overload with impact and vibration.

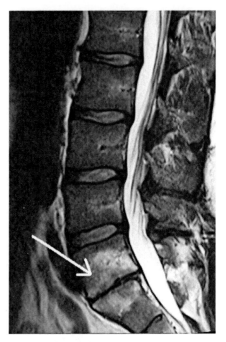

8-3 MRI of isolated disc resorption—arrow points
to degenerative disc—white area around disc is
stress fracturing of trabecular bone

The bone pain is axial low back pain patients describe as "deep, dull, and boring." Many will complain that riding in a car or airplane will set their back off as the disc will not tolerate vibration. Simple prolonged sitting can also be painful, and many patients cannot tolerate sitting through a movie. The pain may have delayed onset for some hours after the triggering activity. Many patients will try to be active but will "pay for it later."

Vibration includes car and bus travel and plane flights. With short exposure, these activities will be disagreeable but normally not intolerable. However, the longer the exposure, the more discomfort will be endured. Impact activities that are very unpleasant include tennis, running, basketball, racquetball, volleyball, football, and skiing. The disc and vertebral body will react typically with dull pain immediately during the activity to a half day later, and severe pain can last twenty-four to forty-eight hours.

The cause of the additional pain is thought to be from nerve fibers in the bone itself. The vertebral bodies are not designed to tolerate significant repeated impact, and small stress fractures occur. These fractures arise in the microscopic bone struts (the trabecula) inside the vertebral bodies. This is the most likely source of the intense, dull pain and why isolated disc resorption is different from the typical back pain from degenerative disc disease. With activity, these fractures become irritated. Swelling and inflammation occur, which renews the pain cycle.

Facet Disease

The facets are the paired joints in the back of the vertebral column. They guide the motion of the lumbar spine. These joints are the same type as knee or hip joints. They have a coating of cartilage and are encased in a capsule that keeps them bathed in lubricating synovial fluid. These joints can develop arthritis just as any others can, and in fact, they tend to become arthritic at a greater frequency. What is unusual is that these joints, even when degenerative, normally do not cause pain. There are however occasions that they do hurt.

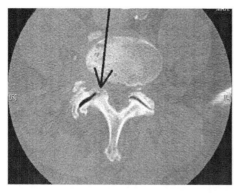
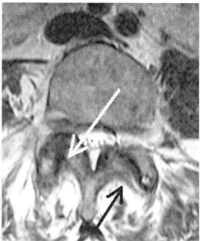

| 8-4A arrow points to degenerative facet | 8-4B MRI of degenerative facet—note white arrow points to slip of the joint |

Facets are loaded when bending backward. Activities that cause extension increase facet pressure and therefore will create pain. The serve or overhead in tennis, swimming, volleyball, and any overhead activity sucwh as painting the ceiling can cause increased pain. Prolonged standing can also aggravate this type of low back pain. If the facets become incompetent (see doorstops in the anatomy chapter), the upper vertebra will slip forward on the one below, causing a degenerative spondylolisthesis that causes different types of symptoms. (See section below.)

Pregnancy and Low Back Pain

Pregnancy by itself causes lower back pain by three different mechanisms. One is that the increased load on the front of the body from the position of the fetus is compensated for by increasing lordosis in the lumbar spine. This increases the load on the facets and causes inflammation and pain. The good news is that when the mother delivers, the load is eliminated, the lordosis normalizes, and the facet inflammation in general disappears.

The other physiological phenomenon that occurs is that the female, when pregnant, secretes a hormone called relaxin. This substance loosens ligaments to allow the pelvis to stretch to accommodate the impending delivery. Ligament laxity can aggravate the overloaded spine to cause pain. Again, delivery normally eliminates the problem.

There is a third category of pregnancy-related back pain that is more problematic. The load on the spine from pregnancy also can occasionally magnify preexisting problems such as a painful degenerative disc, spondylolisthesis, or a herniation. If present, a thorough examination will help uncover one of these pathologies.

Causes Of Leg Pain And Sacroiliac/buttocks Pain

Herniated Disc

This is an extension of degenerative disc disease. The tear in the disc (which itself causes back pain) can finally rip through and through, and the jelly inside (nucleus) can be forced out just like squeezing a toothpaste tube with the cap off. The resultant herniation material pushes against the nerve root, and leg pain ensues.

One of the more interesting scenarios is that in some cases, the patient may have had low back pain for months to years. When the patient lifts or twists, a "pop" occurs in the lower back, resulting in a complete through and through disc tear. Patients will have immediate relief of their long-standing back pain and think they have just won the lottery. This is because the scant remaining intact fibers of the disc were under significant tension. When these fibers rupture, the back pain disappears. This tear of the remaining fibers however allows the nucleus to herniate that compresses the nerve root. Leg pain sometimes takes one to two days to occur after the herniation, so there is a short period of total relief (like the eye of the hurricane).

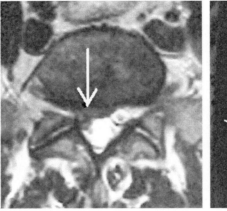 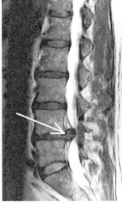

8-5A Herniated Disc—white arrow points to herniation compressing the nerve root

8-5B Large HNP L4-5—arrow points to herniation

Symptoms of a Disc Herniation

If the disc herniation is in the typical posterolateral position, sitting will aggravate sacroiliac and leg pain. Standing or lying down gives some relief. Patients also won't like to bend over to tie their shoes. This holds true if the herniation is at the lower two discs. The reason is that the sciatic nerve is involved. This nerve—a combination of L4, L5, and S1 nerves—travels down behind the back of the pelvis before it descends the leg to "attach" to the foot. When the leg is raised or the patient bends forward, the nerve is stretched over the pulley of the pelvis and pulled into the disc herniation. Buttocks and leg pain become more intense.

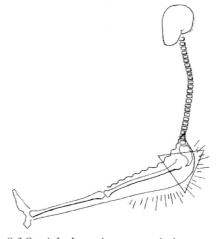

8-6 Straight leg raise test—sciatic nerve
stretched over disc herniation

Now because of anatomy, these rules change if the herniation is at the disc level L3-4 and above. The femoral nerve originates from the roots L2, L3, and L4. Remember, the sciatic nerve is stretched by raising the leg. This motion, however, *relaxes* the femoral nerve. The opposite motion causes the femoral nerve to be stretched. Leg extension (bending the leg behind the body at the hip) pulls on this nerve. The reason is that this nerve travels down the *front* of the pelvis and "attaches" to the front of the thigh and leg. Any backward movement of the leg stretches the nerve over the "pulley" in front of the pelvis and pulls it into the disc herniation.

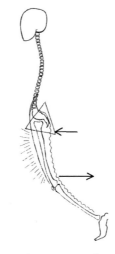

8-7 Femoral nerve stretch—nerve is
compressed against the disc with
leg extension (backwards)

Foraminal Stenosis

Patients with significant narrowing of the hole (or foramen) in the bony spine that the nerve exits through will develop pain down the leg when standing and walking. This is unlike the herniated disc scenario noted above where patients develop pain when they sit. Normally, the longer patients walk with foraminal stenosis, the more pain they develop down the leg. The pain will start in the sacroiliac joint and will radiate farther down the leg the farther they walk. Most almost always feel better when they bend forward, sit, or lie down.

The reason this occurs is that the bony nerve exit hole is made up of a clamshell of the vertebra above and the vertebra below. This outlet is literally made larger by bending forward and narrowed by bending backward. It is also enlarged by leaning away from the painful side and, conversely, made smaller by leaning toward the side of pain. In a normal spine, there is more than enough room for the nerve in this hole no matter what the position of the spine. However, if a bone spur develops, the vertebra collapses on that side from a severely degenerative disc (or rarely a disc herniation occurs in the foramen) that makes this hole narrower the nerve may get pinched. Pain develops over the distribution of the nerve.

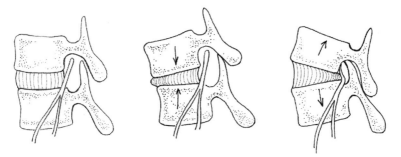

8-8A Flexion—extension changes with foramenal volume

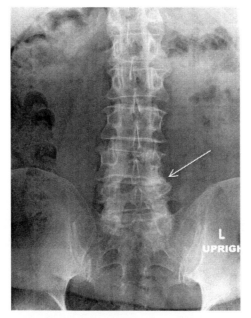

8-8B Foraminal collapse—white arrow points
to L4-5 collapse and angulation

Spinal Stenosis

Spinal stenosis is a variation of foraminal stenosis. Instead of the nerve hole becoming narrowed, the spinal canal where the entire group of nerves resides becomes narrower. Again, like foraminal stenosis, when standing up and walking or especially when bending backward, the canal becomes constricted, and the entire sack of nerves becomes pinched. Symptoms include bilateral buttocks numbness and a heaviness of the legs. These symptoms increase, the more the patient stands and walks and, like foraminal stenosis, improves with bending forward or sitting down. See a more complete discussion of spinal stenosis further in this chapter.

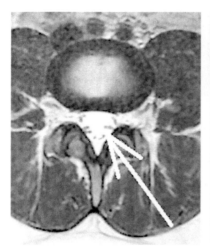

8-9A Normal l MRI—arrow points to spinal canal—black dots are nerve roots floating in white CSF

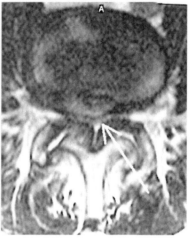

8-9B MRI severe stenosis— white arrow points to nearly obliterated spinal canal

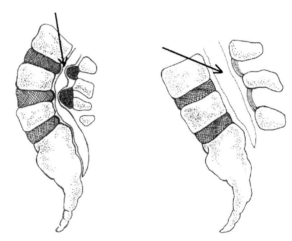

8-9C Flexion extension canal diameter changes—canal becomes smaller with bending backwards

Sacroiliac Joint Dysfunction

The paired sacroiliac joints (SIJ) are strong joints that are composed of both a diarthrodial portion (normal cartilage/synovial joint—like the facet) and a syndesmotic portion (two bones held together by a heavy mass of fibrous tissue). It is rare that these joints become a pain generator. The joints have very little movement and are extremely strong. There is some minor motion in these joints (two degrees) in younger individuals, but as aging occurs, the joints become much stiffer.

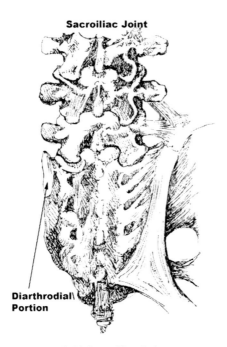

Sacroiliac Joint

Diarthrodial\ Portion

8-10 Sacroiliac Joint

If the joint capsule is torn in front as it commonly is with SIJ pain, inflammation occurs. The structure sitting next to the joint is the sciatic nerve. If this nerve becomes involved in the inflammation mass of the joint tear, pain will radiate down the leg, mimicking sciatica.

The diagnostic physical examination tests for sacroiliac joint disorders are famous and are associated with prominent physicians (Gaenslen's test, Faber's test). They have been around for years and are engrained in treating doctor's psyches. The problem with diagnosis of sacroiliac syndrome is that most of the physical exam tests for this joint are simply inaccurate. Many modern research papers have demonstrated the failure of these tests.

With appropriate injection testing, diagnosis of this joint is relatively simple. An injection into and around the joint with an anesthetic should give good short-term relief (two to three hours). It must be noted that the most common pain that refers to this joint is from irritated nerve roots from the lumbar spine. Many times, the sacroiliac joint is blamed when in reality, it is an innocent bystander.

"Piriformis Syndrome"

The piriformis muscle rests in the back of the thigh under the buttocks. It is a small muscle that traverses the short axis of the thigh from the pelvis to the femur. The sciatic nerve exits the pelvis under it. Occasionally, the sciatic nerve will go right through this muscle. The muscle can have a thick fibrous band within its substance that can occasionally irritate the sciatic nerve.

This muscle has historically been unfairly blamed for the source of many patients' sciatica. The only reason it had been implicated in the past was that it happened to be right in the path of the sciatic nerve. Before the discovery of herniated discs that compress nerve roots, early anatomists used deduction to conclude that the nerve could be compressed by this muscle. This theory made sense as the nerve itself commonly refers pain to this region and will locally be very tender to touch. This syndrome is, however, exceedingly rare and very often overdiagnosed. Most patients with this "syndrome" have nerve pain from the lumbar spine that refers to this muscle.

Cauda Equina Syndrome

This disease is caused by severe compression of the nerves in the spinal canal, normally from a massive herniated disc. This is a surgical emergency and needs to be diagnosed quickly. Without timely decompression of the nerves, permanent damage can occur.

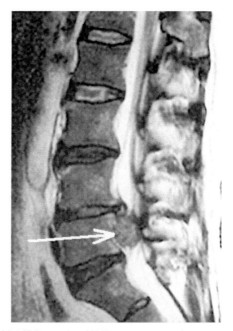

8-11 MRI massive HNP causing cauda equina—
arrow points to herniation

The age of patient is normally in the HNP range (twenty to fifty) but can occur at any age. Pain can be variable, but most patients have severe pain in both legs, with more in the posterior thighs and pelvis. Pain will normally be bilateral. The patient will have sensory loss in the saddle region (inside of the thighs and buttocks) called saddle anesthesia.

The practitioner needs to inquire about bowel and bladder symptoms. Without intact pressure sensation from the bladder, the absent feedback may yield overflow incontinence. The patient's bladder may become so distended and overfilled that the pressure will cause urine to leak out of the urethra without the patient's knowledge. In addition, without the voluntary control of the urinary sphincters, they may not be able to start their flow with intentional urination. Regarding their bowel, they may be constipated, or their sphincter may not work, allowing defecation to occur without their knowledge.

Realize that females who have had children may have had symptoms of bladder leakage for years as the pelvic diaphragm may have stretched out. Cystoceles and rectoceles can develop, causing difficulties with defecation and urination. Older males develop prostate enlargement that makes urination more difficult. Again, a good review of systems will help to ferret out these preexisting symptoms.

Myelopathy

This disease is nicknamed the "Great Imitator." The spinal cord has no pain sensors within its substance. Because of this important fact, there is normally **no pain** associated with spinal cord compression that causes myelopathy. Cord compression normally occurs in the cervical spine, where there will be upper as well as lower extremity symptoms. If compression occurs in the thoracic spine, there will be only lower extremity symptoms.

Symptoms are imbalance in the legs, incoordination in the hands, bowel and bladder dysfunction (normally occurring late in the disease), paresthesias (pins and needles) in the hands and legs, and weakness of the hip flexors (psoas muscle—seen early in the disease). Fine motor skills in the upper extremities suffer such as picking up a dime, buttoning a button, and zipping up a zipper. Handwriting skills may have changed in the last year as hand incoordination makes handwriting sloppier. Balance in a lighted and especially an unlighted room at night may have become worse. Unusual sensations in the arms or legs are not uncommon in myelopathy. Bowel and bladder function may have changed slowly over time. "Lightening"-type sensations down the arms or spine (L'hermitte's sign) with neck flexion or extension are common.

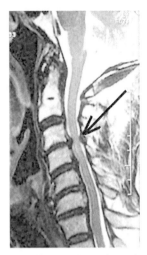

8-12 cervical stenosis and myelopathy

Spinal Conditions That Can Cause Back and Leg Pain

Isthmic Spondylolisthesis (Slipping of a Vertebra Because of a Fracture)

This problem occurs with a fracture in the bone that connects the upper and the lower facets, the pars interarticularis (Latin for "area between the joints"). The break normally occurs because of a stress fracture. This bony area when under stress from athletic activity in extension doesn't have the chance to heal between stressful episodes. Eventually, the stress is greater than the bone can resist, and the area fractures. Since this area of the bone is very poorly supplied with blood, healing is impaired, and the fracture is quite commonly permanent. The most common area for this to occur is L5-S1.

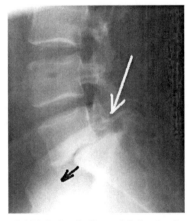

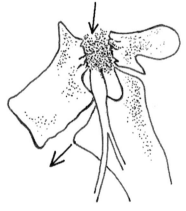

8-13A Isthmic Spondylolysthesis L5—arrow points to fracture

8-13B Isthmic spondylolysthesis— upper arrow points to fracture defect filled with soft tissue

These fractures occur in about one of every twenty adolescents. Normally, the age when this break occurs is quite young—about eight to fifteen years. This defect is more common in athletes that participate in sports that require bending backward (extension) such as gymnastics, diving, volleyball, and football (linebackers). Genetics probably plays a substantial role as 50% of the Inuits (Eskimos) have this fracture.

Symptoms

The fracture almost always starts in children and adolescents. Symptoms that occur when the pars first starts to break varies widely. Some kids actually don't have much pain but only stiffness. If pain does develop, many adolescents will ignore it or won't report it to their parents. Be suspicious of any child that has back pain as to not miss an acute fracture. If these young patients are identified early, they have a chance to heal in a brace.

The unfortunate hallmark of this disorder's symptoms is its variability. As the body tries to heal the fracture, it lays down a number of types of tissues including fibrous tissue, cartilage, and bone. Free nerve endings grow into this mass. This total compilation of bone, cartilage, nerve, and fibrous tissue is called the pannus. This pannus is not as strong as the original pars but can be quite tough and resist tearing for many years. This is why many patients with a spondylolisthesis have no knowledge of this defect and no pain unless the pannus tears.

However, if an abnormally heavy weight or just the right aberrant load stresses the pannus as in a lifting maneuver, the pannus can tear and then become painful. Lower back pain develops. These patients develop symptoms with extension as bending backward loads the inflamed pannus. Some even have pain with flexion as this may stretch the pannus. As you can see, the patient history may become confusing when developing a diagnosis through the history alone.

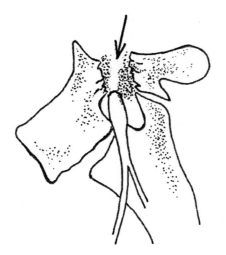

8-14 Isthmic spondylolysthesis—arrow points to
tear in pannus increasing instability and pain

The pedicles where the fractures originally occur can grow spurs as all bony fractures do to attempt healing. These spurs can then become large enough to compress the local nerve roots (L5), and leg pain can eventually develop. Leg symptoms normally increase very slowly over time with pain being intermittent and inconsistent in the beginning. As the spur continues to develop and the nerve hole narrows, leg pain can develop into the majority complaint. The leg pain normally occurs with standing (extension) as this narrows the nerve exit hole and disappears with bending forward or sitting.

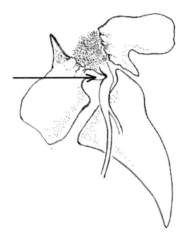

8-15 Isthmic Spondylolysthesis with spur
compressing L5 nerve root—arrow

The vertebral body can slip down the front of the sacrum since the fractured piece of bone is the "doorstop," and the vertebra sits on the sacral slope facing downhill. The actual alignment of the spine can change depending upon the amount of slip since the entire spine follows the L5 vertebral slip. The vertebral slip is noted in "grades." The sacrum is divided into four parts. The first 25% is grade I, from 25-50% is grade II, 50-75% is grade III, 75-100% is grade IV, and if the vertebra slides off the sacrum into the pelvis, this is a grade V or spondyloptosis. Most spondylolisthesis are grade I or II. The higher grades cause significant deformity with the pelvis and upper spine compensating for the slip.

Degenerative Spondylolisthesis

This is a type of slip that occurs when the facet joints (or doorstops) simply wear out instead of break (see facet disease above). Unlike the isthmic spondylolisthesis where the L5-S1 level is the most common, the most common area for a degenerative spondylolisthesis is L4-L5. Most frequently, this disorder occurs in women, but men are not immune to this condition. It is estimated that one in five women will develop this slip by the age of fifty. When these joints wear out and the vertebra slips forward, the spinal canal narrows, and a condition called lumbar spinal stenosis commonly develops.

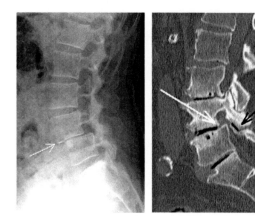

8-16A Degenerative Spondylolysthesis—arrow points to slipped L4 vertebra

8-16B CT scan of degenerative spondylolysthesis—white arrow points to slip of L4 on L5—black arrow points to degenerative facet

Symptoms of Spinal Stenosis

The most common condition that causes this disorder is the slip of a degenerative spondylolisthesis, but stenosis can occur in a "normal" degenerative spine. The lower extremity symptoms normally will start to be noticeable when the nerves are compressed enough to block signals to and from the buttocks and legs.

The constellation of symptoms that develop is called neurogenic claudication. Symptoms increase with standing and walking and are relieved with sitting or bending forward. The classic complaints are that the longer one stands or walks, the buttocks area becomes "achy and numb," and the legs become "heavy." The more prolonged the walking, the more intense the symptoms become until they are intolerable. Finally, the affected individual has to sit down or bend forward, commonly crouching to relieve the pain. After a period of time, the symptoms resolve, and walking can commence again. The cycle then repeats itself.

There is a subset of neurogenic claudication patients who have only lower back pain and no leg symptoms. This particular type of back pain is increased with standing and walking and relieved with bending forward. This is different from patients with degenerative disc disease who get some relief from bending backward and are aggravated by bending forward. For reasons yet to be understood, the pain from neurogenic claudication is only localized and does not radiate down into the buttock and legs.

Mechanics of Spinal Stenosis

The mechanics of this disorder are simple. The spinal canal actually changes in volume with different positions. Bending forward can increase the canal volume by as much as 20%, and conversely, bending backward reduces the capacity by the same amount. It may not be apparent, but the act of walking requires a backward bend of the spine (lordosis). This is done to keep the body over the pelvis to reduce the amount of energy expended while walking. This action reduces the volume of the canal.

Patients with stenosis will unconsciously try to keep their back flat when they walk to keep the canal as open as possible. The only ways to do this are to rotate the pelvis posteriorly and to bend forward. Bending forward while walking wastes a tremendous amount of energy and quickly becomes exhausting. To compensate for this, many patients will keep their knees bent while walking. This maneuver is still very inefficient, but saves more energy than the alternative.

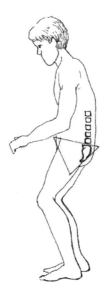

8-17 Stooped forward posture associated with stenosis

Nocturnal Spinal Canal Swelling with Stenosis

Many patients with central stenosis may have increased symptoms in the lower back for about twenty to thirty minutes after getting out of bed in the morning. It may be difficult for these individuals to initially stand upright. This problem is explained by nocturnal swelling of the canal contents at night. The mechanism of this process is easy to understand.

With prolonged standing, many people's ankles will swell because it is the most dependent part of their body. Excess fluid will drain downhill with gravity into the "sump," which with standing or sitting is the ankle region. When these patients sleep, the most dependent part of their body is the lower back, so by default, this region ends up being the sump. Patients with stenosis develop edema in the canal, making the spinal canal more crowded. Standing in the morning will crowd the canal even more until gravity draws the edema out. This makes more room for the nerves, and patients will finally be able to stand up straighter.

Vascular vs. Neurogenic Claudication

Both of these disorders will be associated with similar symptoms and are normally found in the same older patient population. The difference is in how the symptoms manifest. Neurogenic claudication occurs with compression of the spinal nerves. Vascular claudication occurs with deficient blood flow to the muscles of the legs causing build up of lactic acid. Normally both demonstrate bilaterally equal symptoms, but occasionally, neurogenic claudication will be more unilateral. Below is a differential chart of symptoms related to both disorders.

Neurogenic Claudication	Vascular Claudication
Symptoms start proximally and move distally	Symptoms start distally and move proximally
Muscle cramping unusual	Muscle cramping is very common
Relieved by bending forward regardless of activity	No relief with forward bending (unless cessation of activity)
Walking distance prior to onset of symptoms varies day by day	Walking distance always the same prior to onset of symptoms
Riding a bike causes no symptoms	Riding a bike causes symptoms
Continued standing after symptoms develop—no relief of symptoms	Continued standing after symptoms develop—symptom relief

Spinal Malalignment/ Deformity

Scoliosis

Scoliosis is an abnormal curve of the normally straight spine in the frontal plane. Normally, scoliosis should not be painful until the degenerative process advances. The only time the actual nonsymptomatic curve needs to be addressed in a mature individual is when the curve becomes larger or the patient is out of balance. Children with scoliosis are a different story. The curve can silently advance in a child, and treatment commonly is necessary.

In the adult, scoliosis leads to accelerated degenerative changes of the discs and vertebrae. The load on the spinal column is concentrated on a small portion of the total available surface area of the disc and facet. This increased pressure will wear out the segments faster than an evenly loaded spine. A comparison is a car tire knocked out of alignment. Normally, unless you drive like me, you can expect twenty to thirty thousand miles out of a set of tires. However, if the camber is off, the tire will wear in less than five thousand miles as the pressure is increased only on one side of the total potential contact area.

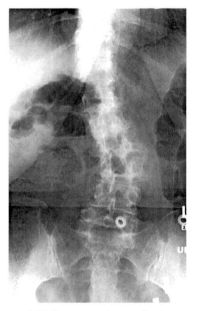

8-18 Degenerative scoliosis

Abnormal Kyphosis

A kyphosis is the name for the curve in the midback (thoracic spine) when an individual is viewed from the side. The normal range for this curve is approximately twenty to forty-five degrees. There are three reasons that this curve can enlarge.

The first is a condition called Scheuermann's disease. Young individuals with this condition have end plates of the vertebrae that become softer than normal. The thoracic vertebra can deform, becoming wedge-shaped, and the thoracic kyphosis can increase, sometimes reaching seventy-plus degrees.

Osteoporosis in the aging spine can cause serial compression fractures that also increase the thoracic curve by causing wedging of the vertebra. Elderly patients may have the "humpback" deformity that is actually a manifestation of this increased kyphosis.

The third cause of increased kyphosis is called postural round back deformity. This condition occurs in adolescents and is a result of very stretchable ligaments, not from deformity of the vertebra.

What do any of these have to do with the lumbar spine? The increased thoracic curve needs to be compensated by the lumbar spine, or the patient will end up with their head pointing at their shoes. The compensation for this condition comes from the lumbar spine in the form of an increased lumbar lordosis.

This increased lordosis can cause increased strain on the facet joints and premature wear. Standing and loading the spine (lifting and impact) will increase low back pain. Muscle overuse pain can also occur with significant malalignment of the back. If the lumbar spine didn't compensate by increasing its curve, the patient would be thrust forward and be out of balance. Increasing the lower back curve requires continuous muscle contraction. This chronic contraction fatigues the muscles, and muscular lower back pain develops. Also involved is chronic contraction of the thoracic muscles that creates muscular midback pain.

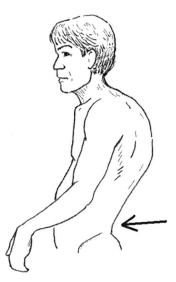

8-19 Scheuermann's hyperkyphosis with
increased lumbar lordosis to compensate

Flat Back Syndrome

The prototypical patient is an older individual with progressive, pan lumbar degenerative disc disease. The patient has lost the normal lumbar lordosis and, therefore, lost their ability to get their torso over their pelvis. This makes them out of balance in the sagittal plane. To compensate and become upright, these patients need to bend their knees to walk. Walking with a flexed knee gait causes significant energy requirements, and these patients fatigue easily. Most prefer to stand holding on to a support such as a cane or shopping cart.

Nonspinal Musculoskeletal Causes

Hip Joint Pathology

Hip disorders can occasionally mimic buttocks and leg pain. The most common region of pain referral occurs in the groin, but a small number of patients will have buttocks pain, thigh pain, and, occasionally, knee pain. The hip joint pain is aggravated with actions like climbing the stairs, getting out of a car, or stepping over an object. The pain can occasionally radiate to the inside of the knee that can mimic a knee problem. If a young child complains of pain on the inside of the knee, the first place to look is the hip. Keep in mind that groin pain can also occur from an L1-3 radiculopathy. The examination is important to differentiate this disorder from radiculopathy.

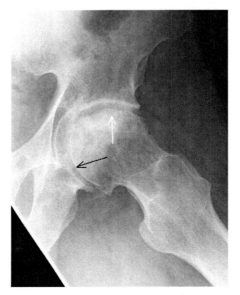

8-20 X-ray of avascular necrosis—black arrow points
to normal region and white to collapsed bone

Tendonitis and Bursitis

Tendons are structures that connect muscles to bone. They insert into the bone through tough tendrils called Sharpey's fibers. These fibers can partially tear under strain, causing pain at this insertion. If either the attached muscle contracts or the tendon is stretched, pain will occur at this insertion point.

A bursa is a synovial fluid-filled sac that is sandwiched between two bones or a bone and a tendon at a high stress point to reduce friction. This area develops friction, and the body's answer is a bursa—essentially, an oil-coated plastic bag sandwiched between the bony prominence and the flat tendon. If the pressure is too great or there is injury to the region of the bursa, it will become inflamed and become thickened. The nerve fibers that surround the bursa become very sensitive, and motion between the tendon and bone becomes painful.

Greater Trochanteric Bursitis

Greater trochanteric bursitis is a cause of lateral hip pain. This condition results from inflammation of the bursa on the outside of the hip joint. It occurs where the large flat tendon of the iliotibial band rubs right on the bony projection off the hip (the greater trochanter). Pain is noted lateral to the hip joint and occurs with hip motion. This bursa can become inflamed and cause local pain, especially with walking or running. Severe inflammation can cause dull local aching even without movement.

Tendonitis of the Ischial Insertion of the Hamstrings

Tendonitis of the insertion of the hamstring muscles into the pelvis (the ischial tuberosity) is rare but can present as buttocks and leg pain. This disorder is essentially tennis elbow of the buttocks. There will be complaints of inferior buttocks pain with passive flexion of the hip (stretching the hamstring) that can radiate down to but not below the knee. Contraction of the hamstrings (active hip extension and knee flexion) will increase the pressure on the insertion and increase pain. Patients have pain that increases with most activities and is relieved with rest. Again, if severe, pain at rest can occur.

Iliopsoas Bursitis

Iliopsoas bursitis occurs in the bursa that overlies the iliopsoas tendon in the groin. Pain will occur with active flexion of the hip such as stair climbing and descending and running.

Peripheral Nerve Entrapment

Any nerve can be entrapped in an area where a nerve traverses a tunnel or a narrow passageway. If the nerve is stretched or inflamed, it swells. A crowded space is just the spot to cause nerve irritability. The nerve will refer pain down its distribution, and if it innervates a muscle, the muscle may become weak. The common places in the leg where a nerve can be entrapped are at the head of the fibula, the groin, and the piriformis muscle in the buttocks. There are entrapment syndromes in the foot, but these shouldn't be mistaken for radiculopathy.

Peroneal Nerve

The common peroneal nerve is a branch of the sciatic nerve. It is exposed at the head of the fibula as it winds its way down the outside of the leg. Compression of this nerve can mimic an L5 radiculopathy with numbness and paresthesias on the dorsum (top) of the foot and foot drop (weakness of the tibialis anterior). There will be no pain radiating from the lower back or buttocks, and position of the spine will not affect the symptoms.

Piriformis—sciatic nerve

As uncommon as it is, piriformis's entrapment of the sciatic nerve deserves to be mentioned. As noted previously, the sciatic nerve travels next to or through a small muscle in the buttocks called the piriformis. On extremely rare occasions, the nerve can be entrapped in the muscle causing sciatica. This is a diagnosis of exclusion as the symptoms will appear to be the same as a radiculopathy of the nerve root. Before this diagnosis is considered, there should be no source of compression found in the spinal area.

Lateral Femoral Cutaneous Nerve

The lateral femoral cutaneous nerve is a sensory nerve that exits into the leg under the inguinal ligament in the anterior pelvis-thigh junction. The nerve's distribution is the anterior and lateral aspect of the leg to but not below the knee. This nerve can be trapped under the ligament and cause pain and sensory disturbance. The symptoms can be misunderstood as an L2 or L3 radiculopathy. There will be no complaints of motor weakness as this is a pure sensory nerve. This nerve can be irritated by wearing a heavy belt (construction workers or police officers) or having Dunlop's syndrome (the belly "done lops" over the belt—a beer belly).

Muscles as the Source of Low Back Pain

There is controversy regarding muscular pain as the root cause of low back pain. Some individuals are convinced that the muscles are one of the main sources of low back pain.

Everyone has had the understanding of what muscular pain feels like. Deconditioned individuals that have performed activities that require repeated muscular contraction have commonly experienced this discomfort. Playing thirty-six rounds of golf or the first day of spring gardening are good examples. The muscles become stiff and achy up to one day later. What happens is that the internal architecture of the muscle becomes disrupted (myosin and actin fibers), and contraction of these muscles is accompanied by pain and dysfunction until the structures become reorganized. Typically, this can take two to three days, but can take as long as one week. These symptoms reflect a classical muscle "strain."

Back disorders are certainly accompanied by muscle spasm, sometimes severe, but the fact is that these spasms with some exceptions are normally the **result** of back instability and not the cause. This, of course, does not mean that treatment is not warranted. These symptoms can be disabling, and treatment in the form of massage is normally very helpful. The root cause of the muscle spasm needs to be discovered and treated, or the massage therapy will only be useful as a short-term therapy.

Muscles *can* generate pain from abnormal biomechanics of the spine (see hyperkyphosis in this chapter). If there is an unstable spinal level, the muscles attempt to stabilize the area by undergoing continuous contraction. The muscles involved build up lactic acid and become stiff and unyielding. Over time, significant muscle pain develops in the area. This pain is relieved by resting the back (sitting in a recliner or lying down). If the pain doesn't dissipate, it probably is not muscle-generated pain.

9

Scoliosis and Kyphosis

Normal Curves—Alignment and Function of the Spine

The vertebrae normally are aligned straight up and down when viewed from the front. An abnormal curve here would be called a scoliosis. From the side, the spine is curved into three C-shaped curves, the normal curves when observed from the side. These are the cervical lordosis, the thoracic kyphosis, and the lumbar lordosis. A lordosis is a curve that angles backward, and a kyphosis is a curve that angles forward. They are all important to the balance of the body. When these curves are functioning correctly, the torso is perfectly balanced over the pelvis. Energy expenditure with walking is minimal, and no pain is noted.

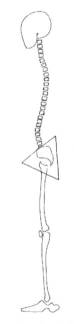

9-1 Normal sagittal alignment

Abnormal Sagittal Curves

Most of the day, gravity pushes our spine forward, and many of our daily activities require forward bending (think computers, reading or writing at a desk, sports such as skiing, cycling, and tennis that all require forward flexion). However, when walking, if the upper body is not positioned directly over the pelvis, the amount of energy necessary to balance the body increases dramatically. This person will fatigue very easily using significant amounts of muscle contraction just to stay upright.

A patient with a sagittal plane deformity will stand with a bent knee, flexed forward posture. This is because in many people, the pelvis cannot normally fully accommodate the loss of lordosis by posteriorly rotating. The only way many individuals use to correct this imbalance is through bending the knees when standing and walking. This will effectively rotate the pelvis backward and help the person to stand upright. The cost of this maneuver is constant contraction of the quadriceps muscle group and greater energy expenditure to stand and walk. It is more efficient however than being bent forward at the waist, contracting the back muscles, and putting the back under significant strain.

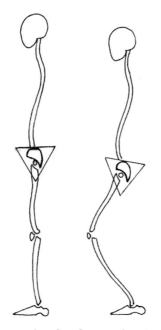

9-2 Compensation for abnormal sagittal curves

Many individuals cannot walk any distance with a bent-knee gait because of knee pain or muscle fatigue, and they must use a walker or cane. This allows the body's weight to be forward and be supported by the reaction force from the ground through the arms using the cane or walker.

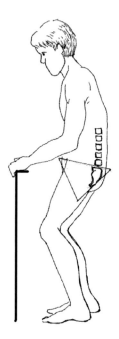

9-3 Cane compensation for anterior sagittal plane deformity

There are four sources for this sagittal plane deformity: antalgia, loss of lumbar lordosis, thoracic hyperkyphosis, and osteoporotic compression fractures.

Antalgic Flat Back Syndrome

The first problem is antalgic posturing, the holding of a posture to prevent pain. The lumbar spine can develop spinal stenosis—a narrowing of the center canal of the spine where the nerves are located. The spinal canal actually changes diameter with different positions. When you bend forward, the canal opens as much as 20% more. When you stand upright, the spine goes into more lordosis, and the canal narrows as much as 20%.

If you already have a lessened diameter to the spinal canal, this closure will compress the nerves and force you either to sit down or bend forward to take the pressure off the nerves. This bent-forward position is called antalgia because it is a posture that you take semiconsciously to get away from pain. You develop a flat back posture to relieve the pressure on the nerves.

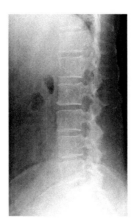
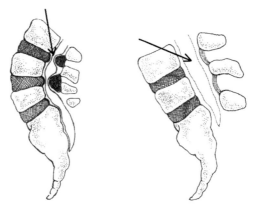

9-4A Lateral standing
X-ray of antalgic
scoliosis from large
herniated disc

9-4B Flexion extension canal diameter
changes—canal becomes smaller
with bending backwards

Loss of Lumbar Lordosis

The second reason for a forward lean from a flat back posture is simple multilevel degenerative disc disease. The reason the lumbar curve is lordotic in the first place is not because of the shape of the vertebrae. Vertebrae are essentially square blocks and, when piled on top of each other, would form a straight column. The curve is the result of the discs that are trapezoidal in shape. When the discs break down, they lose their trapezoidal shape, and this flattens the curve in the back. This is a much more difficult problem to treat because it is a structural problem.

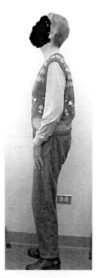

9-5B DDD flat back posturing

Thoracic Hyperkyphosis

The third reason to have a forward lean is from the thoracic spine. If the patient develops an increased thoracic kyphosis from Scheuermann's disease, it will have the same effect as a flattened lumbar spine. The balance of the body is still thrown off in the forward direction, but this time by an increase in the thoracic curve. Accommodation can occur by either increasing the lumbar lordosis or decreasing the sacral inclination.

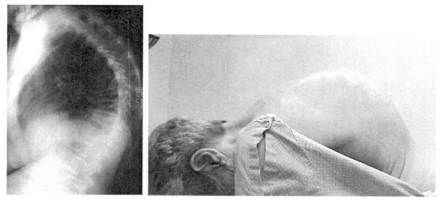

9-6A xray Scheuermann's   9-6B Flexion picture of
kyphosis   thoracolumbar hyperkyphosis

Osteoporotic Compression Fractures

As some patients age and develop osteoporosis, the fractures that occur normally involve the thoracic spine while some also involve the lumbar spine. In either location, the resultant change in alignment will increase the sagittal deformity. This will also increase the load on the remaining vertebral bodies, putting the patient at risk for further fractures.

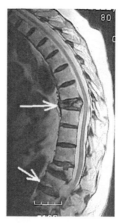

9-7 Thoracic MRI of new and old osteoporosis fractures
with kyphosis—arrows point to new fractures

SCOLIOSIS

Scoliosis is defined as a curve from the frontal plane of greater than ten degrees. Any curve less than ten degrees does not qualify as a scoliosis. There are many different types of scoliosis, each with its own different cause. Some of the more uncommon causes are congenital malformation, neurogenic (cerebral palsy or muscular dystrophy), and paralytic as well as disorders of collagen development (Marfan's syndrome). The three most common types we will talk about are antalgic, idiopathic, and degenerative scoliosis.

Antalgic Scoliosis

An antalgic scoliosis is simply a curve of the back caused by pain and is not a structural deformity. Another name for this compensation is a list. This curve is not structural as when the pain recedes, the curve disappears. These curves are normally caused by nerve root compression and the resultant subconscious "lean" to take the pressure off the nerve. Normally, there is no rotation of the vertebra with an antalgic curve, which is helpful to differentiate it from a scoliotic curve.

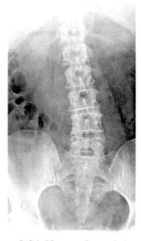

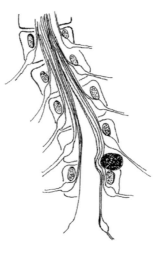

9-8A X-ray of antalgic scoliosis note no rotation of vertebra

9-8B Antalgic scoliosis from disc herniation

Idiopathic Scoliosis

Idiopathic scoliosis occurs in the young population. We don't know the exact cause yet (hence the term "idiopathic"), but we know it is associated with genetic inheritance. Over 10% of first-degree relatives will develop scoliosis. In identical twins, if one has scoliosis, the other has almost a 75% chance of developing it. The prevalence (occurrence in the population) of a curve greater than ten degrees in childhood or adolescence is about two per one hundred individuals. Of curves greater than thirty degrees (much more serious), there is about two per one thousand.

There are three types of idiopathic scoliosis: infantile (ages 0-4), juvenile (ages 4-10), and adolescent (ages 10 to end of growth). Since scoliosis tends to get worse with growth, growth spurts will be particularly hazardous to curve advancement. Especially in adolescence, the growth spurt adds at least two to three inches of overall height gain, and half of this is from the spine. In females, the growth spurt normally occurs about twelve months prior to the onset of menses.

The infantile group is only 0.5% of the total group of scoliosis (90% of these tend to go away [resolve spontaneously]). The ones that don't improve need treatment that is beyond the scope of this book.

Juvenile scoliosis (ages 4-10) is responsible for about 10% of all idiopathic cases. These are more serious as the curves tend to be much bigger. If the curves get to be greater than thirty degrees, these almost always get worse, so treatment is needed. Braces in this group are not very effective, and surgery is required greater than 95% of the time.

Adolescent scoliosis (ages 10 to growth maturity) is responsible for 90% of the scoliosis. Again, only 2% of adolescents have scoliosis, and only 5% of these have curves greater than 30%. Boys and girls have equal occurrences of scoliosis with small curves (ten degrees), but girls have a much greater chance of developing large curves (8:1, girls: boys).

Does scoliosis need to be treated? Curves that end up to be less than thirty degrees normally don't need to be treated. These are relatively stable during adulthood, and most people can live a normal lifestyle without restrictions. Curves greater than forty degrees will typically progress at least one degree per year. Curves in the lumbar spine that are greater than thirty degrees also tend to progress. Advancement of the curve can lead to increased pain in the spine, compression of nerves, and possibly decreased lung function in the largest of curves.

The spinal deformity can also be cosmetically unappealing. Shortened height, a squat stature, and the "rib hump" that occurs in many tend to be seen as unsightly, and the body image that these individuals have can be very displeasing.

Brace treatment can be effective, but you need to understand what the brace can and cannot do. Braces normally don't correct the curve but prevent the curve from getting worse. (A thirty-two-degree curve will normally not turn into a forty-five-degree curve with brace treatment but will also not reduce to a twenty-degree curve when the brace treatment is ended.)

Surgery may be necessary if the curve progresses over forty degrees or progresses in spite of appropriate brace treatment.

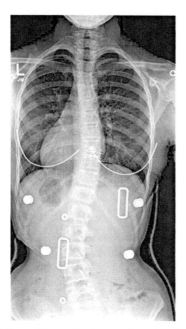

9-9 idiopathic scoliosis—patient in a brace

Degenerative Scoliosis

This curve can occur as a progression from a patient with an old idiopathic scoliosis that is now becoming degenerative or de novo from progressive asymmetric degenerative changes. The treatment rules here are the same as any patient with degenerative changes except that torso imbalance has to be taken into consideration.

10

Inflammatory, Infectious, and Inherited Diseases of Nerves That Cause Leg Pain and Weakness

There are diseases of the nerves that cause leg and arm pain and weakness. These can be divided up into inherited, acquired (developed after birth), and infectious. Nerve diseases cause signals to and from the brain to become interrupted or corrupted, so sensory messages are distorted, the brain can't tell the muscles what to do, and balance is affected. Some of these diseases affect the autonomic system, so "maintenance control" of the body's daily system is affected.

These diseases can also be split up into ones that affect only the peripheral nerves and ones that affect the central nervous system. There are many diseases not mentioned here, but the ones below are the most common ones seen and need to be considered with any spinal diagnosis.

Many of these diseases attack the myelin sheath that surrounds the nerves. To reiterate, the myelin sheath surrounds higher order or more evolved nerves and allows the speed of conduction (the message or signal speed down the nerve) to be very fast. (See chapter on nerve anatomy) The myelin sheath is made of specialized cells called oligodendrocytes (in the CNS) and Schwann cells (in the PNS) that literally wrap themselves around the nerve. Normally, the conduction down the nerve jumps from gaps between these cells (gaps = nodes of Ranvier) significantly increasing the message speed. When these specialized insulation cells are destroyed, the signal slows or stops.

Central Nervous System Diseases

Multiple Sclerosis

This is an autoimmune disease where the body's antibodies attack the myelin sheath of the central nervous system. Females normally outnumber males, 2:1. The disease normally starts between the ages of twenty to forty. The symptoms can start in a variety of locations. Vision loss in one eye, double vision, unusual paresthesias (pins and needles) in the arms or legs, or incoordination, all can be associated with MS. Fatigue and dizziness also are related. The symptoms can be mild or progressive. This disorder is found more often in light-skinned individuals from the northern European countries but can affect anyone. The physical exam (see chapter 18) will demonstrate upper motor neuron findings (hyperreflexia, Hoffman's, clonus, and incoordination)

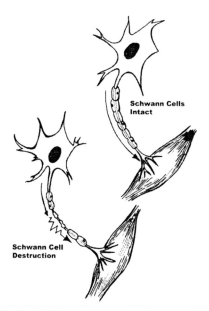

10-1 Multiple Sclerosis—note Schwann cell injury
preventing signal transmission

Diagnosis is important as some treatments can slow down and alter the progress of this disease. Normally, an MRI is used to locate the disease in the brain or spinal cord, and a spinal tap can help with diagnosis.

Polio

This is an infectious disease caused by a virus that attacks the anterior horn cells in the spinal cord. The anterior horn cells are the cell bodies of the motor nerves that connect to the muscles in the arms, the legs, and the diaphragm. Permanent paralysis can occur, and the diaphragm can become paralyzed, requiring a machine to breathe for the patient. Obviously, a vaccine normally confers immunity to this virus, but some parents are now avoiding this vaccine for their children.

Tabes Dorsalis

The sexually transmitted disease syphilis is caused by a spirochete and is normally cured by antibiotics when the first symptoms are noted. If not caught in time, a secondary form occurs, and eventually, a tertiary form that involves destruction of the posterior columns of the spinal cord. The posterior columns are responsible for proprioception (the feeling of position in space). Patients with this disease (tabes dorsalis) walk with a drunken gait as they can't feel their legs when they ambulate. Since the destruction of the spinal cord fibers involves inflammation, this also temporarily increases the output of the brain. Some Middle Ages geniuses who developed great operas, music, or scientific theories were thought to have tertiary syphilis before they went insane from the spirochete destroying their brain.

Peripheral Nervous System Diseases

Peripheral Neuropathy

This is a disease as noted of the peripheral nervous system. It normally starts in the longest nerves (the nerves that go from the spinal cord to the feet), so the symptoms are normally first found in the feet and lower legs. There are many disease processes associated with this disorder. Diabetes, alcoholism, autoimmune diseases, and infectious diseases are some of the causes, but this problem can occur spontaneously.

The symptoms normally start with a "burning numbness" in the feet. Individuals also complain of pins and needles (paresthesias) feelings. The feet can become numb, and walking can be difficult because there is no feedback regarding foot sensation or position. The symptoms can slowly ascend up the legs, and the upper extremities can eventually be involved. When the hands become involved, it is known as a "stocking and glove" involvement. This process can affect the motor nerves too, but this disease process mainly affects the sensory nerves. The symptoms seem to be intensified at night, making sleeping difficult. Some patients have allodynia—hypersensitive feet and cannot tolerate the weight of a simple bedsheet.

Treatment involves both symptomatic relief as well as taking care of the process that caused this neuropathy in the first place. With diabetes, making sure the sugar levels are kept in a tight range is important. With alcoholism, obviously stopping the use is paramount. For symptomatic relief, the membrane stabilizers (see pharmaceutical chapter) can work well. Shoes that fit well and are not tight are mandatory.

Guillain-Barré Syndrome

This disease is also known as ascending paralysis. It occurs days to weeks after a viral infection. Again, it is an autoimmune disorder. It starts with weakness in the legs and ascends up, normally in a matter of weeks, but there are known cases that had ascended in only three to four hours. In its mildest form, the symptoms of GBS may only be fatigue and not be recognized. The problem is that it can ascend to the diaphragm level and prevent breathing. The patient would have to be put on life support until the disease process abates.

The effects of the disease normally disappear within months. Fifteen percent of patients, however, have lasting physical impairments.

Charcot-Marie-Tooth Disease

This is an inherited disease of peripheral nerves. Its other name is "peroneal muscle atrophy." Here, the myelin sheath is diseased, and also the nerve itself is involved. This syndrome affects both motor and sensory nerves. Its hallmark is a cavovarus foot with clawing of the toes. That is, a very high arch, a turned in foot with arched toes. There is also in some individuals a "stork leg" appearance. The muscles of the lower leg atrophy, but the upper leg muscles stay intact, giving a bird leg (stork leg) look. Ten percent of CMT patients have spinal deformities. Intrinsic muscles can also be involved.

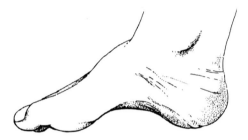

10-2 Charcot Marie Tooth foot changes—
high arch and claw toes

Amyotrophic Lateral Sclerosis (ALS or Lou Gehrig Disease)

This is a disease of only peripheral motor nerve cells causing their death. It causes wasting of the involved muscles. What makes this disease different is that the sensory system is spared. Loss of strength, weakness, and clumsiness are the initial symptoms. The muscles exhibit fasciculations (nonpurposeful twitching) that differentiate it from myelopathy and other neurological diseases. As the disease progresses, speaking, swallowing, and even breathing become difficult. Patients normally succumb to respiratory diseases.

Lyme Disease

This is an infectious neurological disease caused by the organism *Borrelia burgdorferi*, a spirochete. It is transmitted by the bite of a small tick. There is a time period between the tick bite and disease onset of three to thirty-two days (incubation period). In 80% of individuals, they will exhibit erythema migrans. As the name implies, a small area of redness (macule or papule) spreads into a large red ring with central clearing (like a target). There can be headaches, fevers and chills, muscle pain, and fatigue in this stage.

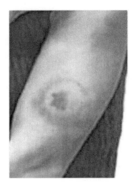

10-3 Lyme disease target lesion

Fifteen percent will develop frank nerve abnormalities including meningitis, encephalitis, cranial neuritis (Bell's palsy), plexitis, and mononeuritis multiplex.

Months to years later, the patient will manifest chronic nerve manifestations. They can develop changes in mood, memory, and sleep. Some will have spinal and radicular pain. Eight percent will get cardiac involvement.

This disease is treated with a simple antibiotic (doxycycline) if caught early.

Herpes Zoster (Shingles)

As most of you know, this is caused by the same virus that causes chicken pox. Once the virus varicella has waned in symptoms, the virus lies dormant in a dorsal root ganglion of a spinal nerve. Much later, the virus is activated by an unknown type of stressor. The first symptom is pain down the dermatome of the nerve. The typical rash occurs two to three days later. The rash appears as small reddened fluid-filled blisters (vesicles) that increase for the next three days before they finally dry up. Small scars may occur. The symptoms are normally unilateral (one sided) and occur more frequently in the chest area but can occur anyplace including the arm or leg. If the patient develops postherpetic neuralgia (painful scarring of the nerve), this is a permanent chronic painful condition of the nerve. Treatment with a steroid during the attack may prevent nerve scarring.

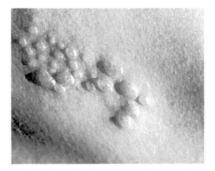

10-4 Rash of Shingles—note the vesicles and
macules along a dermatome

11

Rheumatological Conditions (Spondyloarthropathies)

These problems are not associated with the typical degenerative conditions that are seen day to day in the clinic. The "normal" conditions that are seen every day are caused by the genetics of weaker collagen, the wear and tear of everyday activities, and any trauma that we experience.

Rheumatological problems are due to autoimmune disorders of the musculoskeletal system. Our own immune system goes haywire. Normally the parts of the immune system become triggered by various alien proteins such as those from bacterial or viral origin. For various reasons, the immune system can become confused and see parts of our own indigenous protein as foreign invaders. It then goes about its duty of rejecting these "foreigners" by attacking the very structures it is designed to protect. When the immune system mistakenly identifies a natural protein in the spine as "foreign," inflammation, swelling, erosion of bone, and joint and nerve destruction can occur.

Symptoms of Autoimmune Spinal Disorders

Except for rheumatoid arthritis, most spinal autoimmune diseases start with sacroiliac joint involvement. Some of these diseases that involve the SI joint attack both sides, but most are unilateral. The classic first symptom is stiffness in the morning that goes away with activity. Stiffness that goes away with exercise is the sine qua non for spinal autoimmune disorders. Fatigue is also a harbinger of symptoms of the disease.

Rheumatoid arthritis, psoriasis, ulcerative colitis and Crohn's, Reiter's syndrome, ankylosing spondylitis, lupus, myositis, polymyalgia rheumatica, and DISH are some of the diseases associated with spine pain and stiffness.

X-ray Findings

X-rays have some classic findings for these disorders. Syndesmophytes are bone spur formations that occur off the upper and lower end plates of the vertebral bodies.

They can be categorized as marginal and nonmarginal. Marginal syndesmophytes are spurs that originate immediately out of the body and connect one vertebra to another through the "margin" of the vertebra. Marginal syndesmophytes stay within the confines of the anterior and posterior longitudinal ligaments and are pathonomonic for ankylosing spondylitis. The spine has the appearance of segmented bamboo, so it is called a "bamboo spine." Nonmarginal syndesmophytes normally occur with psoriasis, ulcerative colitis, Crohn's, Reiter's syndrome, and DISH.

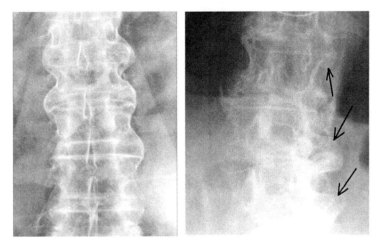

11-1A Bamboo spine from ankylosing spondylitis

11-1B Claw or parrot beak osteophytes associated with spondyloarthopathies

Sacroiliac joints are the first joints to be involved with many of these disorders. By simple x-ray, these joint's involvement can be difficult to diagnose. The edges may become blurred, and occasionally, the joint actually fuses and disappears on x-ray. If the joint is involved, bilateral involvement is ankylosing spondylitis, and unilateral involves most of the others.

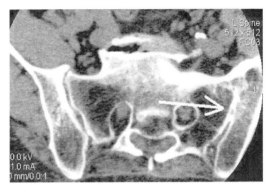

11-2 CT scan of sacroiliac autofusion arrow points to autofusion

Rheumatoid arthritis (RA) is a destructive disease that can be obvious on x-ray. RA destroys the synovial joints, so the vertebral bodies look normal, but the facets become eroded. C1-2 has a synovial joint between the dens and the arch of C1. The disease can therefore cause a larger gap on the lateral cervical x-ray between C1 and C2. Commonly, degenerative spondylolisthesis of the lower vertebra occurs with this disease process, and the cervical spine is affected much more commonly than the lumbar spine.

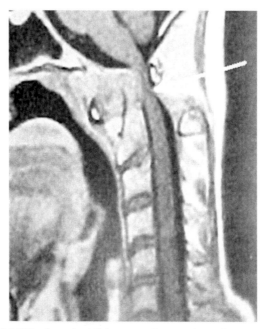

11-3 MRI of cervical RA—note destruction of transverse
ligament and cord compression—white arrow

Rheumatoid Arthritis (RA)

This disease attacks the synovium lining the joints over parts of the body. Since the spine has synovial joints (the facets and the C1-2 joints at the base of the skull), it is not immune to this disorder. The disease typically involves the joints of the hand at an early stage. Swelling and pain of the finger joints signal the onset. RA is symmetrical. That is, if the left fingers are involved, the right ones will be too. Nodules will form underneath the skin that can be painful.

The disease also affects other body parts such as the blood vessels (vasculitis) and the nerves. Mononeuritis multiplex looks like unrelated multiple occurrences of a single nerve involvement (the tibial nerve on the left and the median nerve on the right stop working normally). What is happening is the vascular supply to the nerve is cut off, starving the nerve of oxygen.

The lungs can be affected as well as the lining of the heart.

You would think that with such a well-known disease such as rheumatoid arthritis, there would be one test to determine if a patient has it. That is not the case. Some of the tests such as rheumatoid factor show up in 3% of healthy population. It is estimated that 1-2% of the population has rheumatoid arthritis.

When it affects the spine, the neck is the most affected. Only rarely does the thoracic or lumbar spine become affected. The symptoms almost always start with stiffness and decreased range of motion of the neck.

Seronegative Spondyloarthropathies

These are potentially related diseases that do not have a blood test to help with the diagnosis—hence the term "seronegative" (the serum tests are negative). They have many features in common, such as the involvement of only one side of the sacroiliac joint that can go on to fuse, nonmarginal syndesmophytes (discussed earlier in this chapter), and fatigue/lethargy. Many of the patients have a finding on a chromosome called the HLA—B27 gene. However, just like rheumatoid arthritis, this gene is found in the normal population, so it is not diagnostic by itself. The diseases are enteropathic arthritis, psoriatic arthritis, and Reiter's syndrome.

Morning stiffness is the hallmark of spondyloarthropathies. Don't forget that morning stiffness is also associated with DDD and stenosis. Patients with all three diseases feel somewhat better with a shower and some stretching, but the patient with spondyloarthropathy will feel significantly better. Where the DDD patient will have increased symptoms with exercise, the spondyloarthropathy patient will tolerate the workout without significant problems. Sacral or axial lumbar pain will be present in both. Spondyloarthropathy is not normally associated with leg pain where DDD can be. Reiter's patients however may complain of heel pain.

Ankylosing Spondylitis

The prototype for autoimmune spinal disorders is ankylosing spondylitis. This is a disease process where the spine literally fuses itself over time. Found generally in younger males, it has some classic symptoms called the prodrome where the actual disease process may not be identified for months after the initial symptoms. It is estimated that one in every thousand Caucasians has this disease. Females can also succumb to AS. The blood marker HLA-B27 is common with this disease. Its presence does not absolutely indicate disease, and its absence does not ensure the lack of disease.

Young adult males will develop morning stiffness and a pain in the lower back (sacroiliac involvement). Sleep can be difficult. Some will develop iritis, an inflammation of the anterior chamber of the eye. This disease is cyclical. That is, it is noted for exacerbations and remissions. Again, think ankylosing spondylitis if there is morning stiffness that gets better with activity in a young adult male.

Reiter's Syndrome

Reiter's is associated with either a sexually transmitted disease called chlamydia or can be noted occasionally with a bacterial infection of the intestines. Sometime after the infection ceases, the syndrome begins. The triad consists of urethritis, conjunctivitis, and arthritis (inflammation of the urethra, the eye, and the joints). The syndrome consists of heel pain and swelling, probably from an inflammation of the insertion of the Achilles tendon or plantar fascia, back pain from the sacroiliac joint, and inflammation of the eye.

Conjunctivitis occurs in 40% of patients, and sacroiliac involvement occurs in 70% of patients. Myalgias can occur (pain in the muscles themselves), and a very swollen finger (sausage digit) also is seen with Reiter's syndrome.

Psoriatic Arthritis

Psoriasis is primarily known as a skin disease. The skin on extensor surfaces (normally the elbows and knees) becomes reddened and develops a silvery scale. A small percentage of these patients develop arthritis. Psoriatic arthritis and spondyloarthropathy is associated with changes in the nail beds on the fingers. The condition called "sausage digits" can be noted in some where the involved digit enlarges markedly.

If a patient with psoriasis develops arthritis, 95% have peripheral joint involvement (elbows, knees, and hips), and 5% have spinal involvement including the typical nonmarginal syndesmophytes.

Enteropathic Arthritis

"Enteropathic" refersto the intestines. The two diseases commonly known are Crohn's disease and ulcerative colitis. Both involve intestinal debilitation, and both are known to involve the spine. Ten to twenty percent of patients will develop sacroiliitis or sacroiliac involvement, and 10% will develop spondylitis or spinal inflammation.

Myalgias and Fibromyalgia

Myositis and Myalgias

There are some unusual diseases that cause muscle-generated pain such as polymyalgia rheumatica and myositis. These are systemic autoimmune diseases related to temporal arteritis. In these cases, the immune system stops recognizing the muscles as "self" and starts attacking them. Patients with this problem have debilitating muscle aching. The common flu also causes generalized muscle pain (myalgias) by a similar mechanism.

Fibromyalgia

Fibromyalgia is a controversial diagnosis as there are no lab tests, x-rays, or other concrete ways to prove this diagnosis exists. The only way to make this diagnosis is to exclude any other potential diagnoses and inventory the patient's complaints to see if these fit with fibromyalgia guidelines.

The most common patient is a female of childbearing years. This syndrome tends to get somewhat better with activity, but most patients will have not engaged in exercise. The patients complain of stiffness and lethargy. Headaches, irritable bowel syndrome, and sleep disturbances are quite common. This disorder is commonly associated with depression, so the four depression questions need to be asked to discover if depression is present. To diagnose this disorder, there needs to be pain in all four quadrants of the body—legs, arms, pelvis, and central core—with eleven of eighteen tender points present in specific areas. Treatment is similar to chronic pain syndromes.

12

Osteoporosis

The human body needs calcium in the blood for normal activity. Many women and some men, as they age, lose calcium from the bone into the blood. The bone gets thinner and more prone to fracture. The bone can get so soft that a simple step off a curb can cause a fracture of the spine.

Once the bone becomes brittle enough and fractures occur, these fractures can become catastrophic. A stumbling fall causing a hip fracture in the elderly can be surgically fixed easily enough, but the chance of surviving six months after the hip fracture is significantly diminished. Vertebral fractures cause pain and spinal deformity. Normally, they occur in the thoracic and lumbar spines. When fractures occur, they can cause a significantly increased kyphosis in the thoracic spine or decreased lumbar lordosis, both causing increased sagittal plane deformity. Fractures can occasionally cause compression of the nerves and spinal cord.

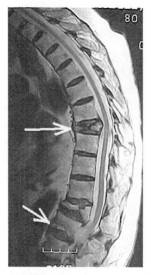

12-1 Thoracic MRI of new osteoporosis fractures
with kyphosis—arrows point to new fractures

To diagnose osteoporosis, a bone density scan is used. This passes a predetermined amount of an x-ray beam through a specific area of the body, normally a hip, lumbar spine, and wrist. The amount of beam blocked indicates the density or "thickness" of the bone. Comparisons to normals give a "T" score. A certain lower score would be osteopenia, and a lower score than that would be true osteoporosis.

There are new oral and injectable treatments for osteoporosis. These prevent the calcium from the bone from being removed by the osteoclasts.

Treatment of Osteoporotic Fractures

Many osteoporotic fractures can be treated as simple compression fractures. A brace and tincture of time and the fracture will generally heal well. This may leave some deformity (angulation of the spine), but most of the time, the deformity is minimal, or the patient adapts well to go on with their life.

If there is considerable pain and deformity, a newer technique has been developed to help reduce these problem fractures. This procedure is called vertebroplasty or kyphoplasty. Through a minimal skin incision, a small balloon is introduced into the fractured body of the vertebra. The balloon is expanded to create a space where the vertebra had collapsed and then filled with polymethyl methacrylate as a spacer. This is the same cement used to put in artificial hips and knees. This procedure seems to immediately reduce the spine pain and help with the deformity in many patients. The long-term effects of the cement are still not known in this area, but this same cement has been used in hip and knee joints with good longer-term success.

Scoliosis

The problem with osteoporosis in the spine is twofold. One is it may lead to compression fractures, and the second is with scoliosis. With scoliosis, the spine is loaded asymmetrically. If the bone becomes weaker, it will fail on the inside curve of the spine where the pressure is greater. This makes the scoliosis curve greater, putting even more stress on the already stressed bone. This could lead to even greater chances of the vertebra fracturing and the curve advancing. Without scoliosis but with a significant angulation of the spine in the sagittal plane from the fracture or fractures, the bending moment force on the spine becomes greater. This puts the spine at greater risk for further fractures.

13

Dangerous Mimics of Disc Pain

Pain in the lumbar spine does not have to originate from the spine itself. There are many referral structures that can cause low back pain and need to be ruled out as a source of pain.

To understand why some of these structures would cause low back pain, we have to go back to embryology. The structures in the retroperitoneum (the area behind the intestines) are supplied by the same nerve endings as the back structures. Sometimes, the brain has difficulty differentiating where pain comes from in this area. These structures include the aorta, kidneys, pancreas, gallbladder, urinary bladder, ovaries, and uterus. Any problem with one of these organs could refer pain to the back.

The most devastating one is an abdominal aortic aneurysm. The aorta is the main artery that brings blood to the lower body. It travels next to the spine in the abdomen. Occasionally in individuals older than sixty with high blood pressure or genetic diseases, the aorta can stretch out, and pain from this can refer to the back. The danger is that this vessel can rupture, and surgical repair can be lifesaving if done in time.

Kidney infections are famous for referring pain to one side of the back, where the ribs meet the lower back. This is called costovertebral tenderness and is elicited by percussing at the lowest ribs alongside the spine. Severe pain in this region can be an indicator of a kidney infection.

Gynecological problems can refer pain to the back. Endometriosis and ovarian cysts are two good examples. This pain will normally be cyclical with the patient's period. A pelvic infection from any number of causes can also cause pain. Ectopic pregnancy, a surgical emergency, can refer to the back. It is important to get a thorough history of the patient's cycles and activities to help rule this in or out.

Occasionally, diverticulitis can cause back pain. This occurs when small outpouchings of the intestinal wall become inflamed.

Gallbladder attacks can cause back pain. Normally, these would be worst after a fatty meal and are crescendo-decrescendo (get worse and then better in a matter of minutes) type of attacks. That is, the pain rises and falls as a crampy type of pain.

Cancer can obviously cause back pain. If a vertebra or pelvis fractures because the bone is weakened, the pain will be like typical fracture pain. X-rays and especially an MRI would differentiate this. Compression of a nerve or the cauda equina will give symptoms associated with these specific structures.

Infection of the spinal column—discitis or osteomyelitis is always a concern and has to be kept in the differential diagnosis. Many patients may not have constitutional symptoms such as fever, chills or even significant back pain. Many will have muscle spasms, malaise and some will present with an ileus (intestinal obstruction) as the first sign of a spinal infection. Interestingly, some will have a low grade temperature or even be normal. Lab studies are frequently abnormal (ESR and CRP) but I have seen some patients with osteomyelitis and normal labs. An MRI is the test of choice if you are concerned.

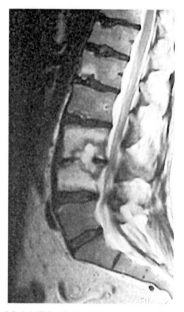

13-1 MRI of discitis-osteomyelitis
of the L3-4 disc space

14

Treatment of Mechanical Lower Back Disorders

This chapter is devoted to the types of mechanical and medicinal therapies to help improve pain and dysfunction from various spinal disorders. The first step is the diagnosis of the disorder as this will dictate what therapies can be useful. The next step is the understanding of the biomechanics of the disorder. The last step is how to reverse or ameliorate the problem mechanics and strengthen the associated muscles. This is essence of therapy.

This chapter is not a cookbook. It does not give advice on how many repetitions of what specific exercise needs to be done to strengthen what particular muscle. This section explains the biomechanics, gives guidelines on what mechanical changes need to be done to alter the stresses and the general way to do it. As has been noted, a skilled and knowledgeable therapist, no matter what the specialty, is one of the keys to pain relief and better function.

Medications can be used to reduce inflammation, reduce pain, relax muscles, and calm nerves. Pharmaceuticals can also be used for reactive depression and sleep disorders related to pain. This chapter will just touch on their use, but the chapter on medications will be more helpful.

General Considerations

In general, what can be done with rehabilitation? Therapists can educate patients to strengthen and condition muscles, stretch ligaments and discs, and learn better mechanical ways of doing activities (ergonomics). Cardiovascular training also plays a large part in recovery. Muscle strengthening is designed to make the muscle capable of supporting a heavier load. Conditioning makes the muscle more resistant to fatigue from repeated stress. Stretching can reduce and alter loads to spinal structures, and ergonomics is a way to retrain the body to lift, bend, and load the spine that reduces stress. Restrictions sometimes are in order to prevent painful and destructive loading of the spine.

In sports, there are adjustments to be made to the bike, skis that are designed to be more impact tolerant and binding setting that can be more forgiving. There are shoes that can reduce shock and some sports that may just simply need to be avoided. Hikers can use ski poles to unload the spine. Athletes can change their form to minimize impact and torsion.

All individuals can strengthen their cardiovascular system (heart and lung conditioning). No matter what the disorder is, cardiovascular training has been demonstrated to significantly help with pain reduction as well as allowing muscles to work longer without becoming fatigued. This is a cornerstone for spinal rehabilitation, and not enough emphasis is put on this training.

Core Strengthening

If there is one key phrase used to describe back pain rehabilitation, it is to "strengthen the core." The reason core muscles are so important is that they are one of the major keys to stabilize the spine no matter what the diagnosis. Every single disorder found in this chapter will benefit from core strengthening. Discs can't be made stiffer any other way unless the patient undergoes surgery or awaits Father Time for further degenerative changes. The core muscles can be strengthened to help control the abnormal motion of the disc. Please see chapter 4 for the anatomy of this group of muscles.

Think of the lumbar spine as bunch of loosely joined building blocks. The muscles that *directly* insert into these blocks are small and generate poor strength. That is, they can't generate the necessary forces to restrain abnormal movements of the spine. The long (and strong) extensor muscles of the back don't directly attach into the lumbar spine vertebra, so they can't individually affect stability. They do however attach into all the surrounding structures to give group (or core) stability.

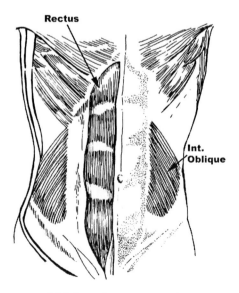

14-1 Anterior core muscles

To make the elbow stiff when holding a heavy object, contraction of the front muscle of the arm (triceps) stabilizes the joint. The opposing muscle is reflexively inhibited to prevent damage to the joint (reciprocal inhibition). This is different from the spine. When the core is strong, muscles actually work against each other to stop motion of the spine, essentially "splinting" the spine. Contraction of the anterior wrapping and posterior muscles at the same time immobilizes the core by increasing the abdominal pressure through the anterior muscles. Also, compression of the thoracic spine onto the pelvis occurs with the posterior extensor muscles. The abdominal contents act like a giant water balloon wrapped by a boa constrictor. Contraction of the abdominal muscles increases pressure in the belly that is opposed by the pelvic floor and the diaphragm in turn that stiffens the lumbar spine even more.

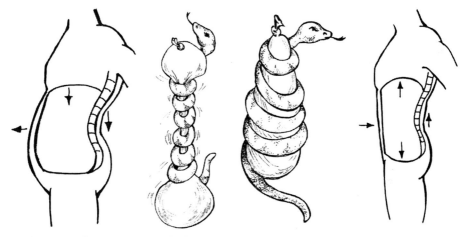

| 14-2A Weak core muscles—increased lumbar lordosis and increased stress on discs | 14-2B Snake compressing water balloon elongates balloon | 14-2C Strong core muscles—increased abdominal pressure distracts and stiffens spine reducing pressure on discs |

One important fact: muscle strengthening takes time for results to occur. The differences from week to week are not easily noticeable, and the progress can be frustrating. Patience and the consistency of performing these exercises are the basis to increasing strength and stability. At least two and probably three months of strengthening with unswerving work on the core will be needed before a noticeable difference can be seen.

Strength without Injury

Any muscle can be strengthened with the appropriate amount of work. One of the keys is to strengthen muscles without hurting the structures they protect. Anyone can go to the gym, get involved in an aerobics class and weight room, and gain strength and endurance. If that individual has a symptomatic disc or a spondylolisthesis, however, many exercises will be painful. A patient will be discouraged by performance training they think will be beneficial, only to have increased pain after the exercises. This is where a good therapist comes in. A well-trained therapist can design a program that will not be harmful and still lead to strength and conditioning.

Lever Arms and Archimedes' Principle (Ergonomics)

One of the problems with the lower back muscles is that they are at such a mechanical disadvantage. If we look at a simple diagram of spinal biomechanics, remembering basic physics and principles of lever arms, the force generated by bending forward and lifting has to be resisted by an exact opposite force. This opposing force is generated by the pull of the back muscles and the dampening restraint of the ligaments and discs.

As may appear obvious, you can see that the heavier the load, the more stress occurs to the lower back. What is not immediately obvious is that the farther away the load is from the body, the more stress is generated to the back. Also, the more bent forward, the more Archimedes' principle of lever arms comes into play. The torso and upper extremities are the lever arm, and the farther the individual bends forward, the longer the lever arm and, therefore, the greater the strain on the back.

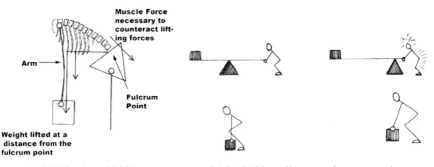

14-3B Physics of Lifting   14-3A Lifting diagram demonstrating
                                     increased stress with loading further away

This is where ergonomics plays an important role. The simple act of lifting can be made much less damaging to the spine by bringing the load much closer to the body and keeping the back flat while bending the knees. Use the knees to lift as the quadriceps muscles are very strong.

Avoid Bacon, Lettuce, and Tomato (BLT)

There are many positions that can load the spine that are not healthy for the discs. The discs "abhor" rotation (twisting or lateral bending) as it puts them at a mechanical disadvantage. When one twists, 50% of the fibers of the disc are relaxed, and the other 50% are put under significant load. Then, with a forward bend, all the tension is put on the posterior part of the disc that further increases the stress on the already overloaded fibers. Combine a twisting motion with a forward bend and then a lift, and a perfect environment for an annular tear has been created.

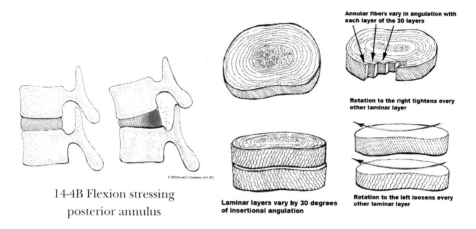

14-4B Flexion stressing posterior annulus

Annular fibers vary in angulation with each layer of the 30 layers

Rotation to the right tightens every other laminar layer

Laminar layers vary by 30 degrees of insertional angulation

Rotation to the left loosens every other laminar layer

Unfortunately, many people lift this way. This is a learned behavior as this is the easiest way to move an object with the least expenditure of energy (but the most strain on the back). This is all fine and good if the individual is young and the disc is resistant to tear, but with any aging or genetic predisposition, this is a recipe for injury. Patients have to *relearn* how to lift to avoid this position (the BLT position—**B**ending and **L**ifting when **T**wisting).

General Modalities to Work on Inflamed Tissue

The chiropractor or therapist may have different types of devices to help reduce swelling and inflammation. These are ultrasound, electrical muscle stimulation, TENS and high-current TENS, diathermy, and traction. Some therapists may have access to iontophoresis.

Ultrasound works by inducing high-frequency sound waves into tissues. This will cause the molecules in the tissue to vibrate quickly, inducing heat into the tissue. Ultrasound is useful for inflamed tissues such as muscles or bursa. Electrical muscle stimulation causes the muscles under the surface pads to contract. This is useful for the later stages of injured muscles and can reduce fatigue of muscles. TENS is covered in the alternative chapter but is a surface stimulator that reduces local pain. Diathermy induces local heat into the tissue. Traction is useful for the cervical spine but much less useful for lumbar disorders. Iontophoresis is the use of current to drive medications under the skin. It can be used on a pad that produces its own current or be driven in by an ultrasound/current combination.

Pilates

This book is not designed to endorse any specific program as a great therapist may come from many different types of schools. However, if there is one set of exercises that is generally helpful in most situations, it is "Pilates." These series of exercises are some of the most consistent endeavors to achieve a strong core. Mind you, there are many other techniques that can also strengthen the core, and an uneducated Pilates instructor can do more harm than good.

MedX Treatment

The MedX is a machine designed to activate and exercise the small extensors of the back. In a normal exercise routine, only the large muscles of the spine are significantly activated. This machine essentially isolates the small intervertebral muscles and strengthens them. It does so by mechanically locking the pelvis and using a series of counterweights to offset and neutralize the weight of the torso. True back extensor strength can also be measured. This device is truly an exercise machine, so it is not an alternative treatment per se, but since it is uncommon to be used, it is included in this chapter. This treatment apparatus is normally found in a physical therapist's office or a chiropractor's office as an adjunct and can be very effective.

Treatment of Specific Diagnoses

Annular Tears

This is an acute injury. It may seem like a simple "give" in the lower back at the time, but if there is an inflammatory response, the patient may be incapacitated. With a simple tear, the symptoms will disappear within two days to as much as six weeks and, generally, will cause no further problems. This is called a self-limiting injury as it will generally fade away with time. There are treatments that can reduce the symptomatic period.

A back brace or corset makes the patient comfortable. Physical therapy modalities such as electrical muscle stimulation, massage, and ultrasound can reduce the spasms. Chiropractic manipulation, if done carefully, can also reduce spasm. Medications such as painkillers, NSAIDs, and muscle relaxants are helpful. With severe pain and spasm, consideration of a short-term oral steroid should be given. Obviously, significant reduced activity goes hand in hand with severe pain and spasm. One to two days of bed rest may be in order at the severe onset of pain but should be avoided as soon as the patient can ambulate. Epidural injections in the most symptomatic cases can be helpful, but this may require an MRI prior to the injection.

Degenerative Disc Disease

The key for treatment of degenerative disc disease is to think in terms of management. As has been noted before, discs don't heal, so self-care needs to be a lifetime affair. This is actually not as much a perceived problem as it seems as a successfully managed patient will be stronger and fit. If the home exercises don't become habit however, eventually the muscles become weaker, old bad routines will rear their ugly heads, and the symptoms may reappear.

For acute flare-ups, the same treatment as an annular tear noted above is in order. For chronic symptoms, stretching, strengthening, and conditioning are important. Stretching is importantly to perform slowly. A slow, gentle, continuous stretch is more therapeutic than a bouncing-type stretch. In general, degenerative discs won't become more mobile with stretching (that would not be beneficial), but improvement of the motion of the surrounding discs will improve that in turn takes the stress off the painful one.

Hamstring muscles are commonly tight with degenerative disc disease, and this tethers the pelvis. Tethering the pelvis makes it unable to act as a shock absorber, and the lumbar spine sees more stress. An absolute to reduce spine discomfort is to stretch the hamstrings every night until the patient can come close to touching the toes.

As will be repeated ad nauseam in this chapter, core strengthening is the key to improvement and pain relief. The core muscles are the best way to splint the lumbar spine and reduce stress on the discs. Start with pure isometrics for a much deconditioned core (strengthening with no motion of the spine) and advance to isotonics (strengthening with motion) when the muscles have developed some endurance and resistance.

Medications can be very helpful. The list is similar to annular tear treatment protocol, but oral steroids are not used unless there is a severe flare-up. Narcotic medications need to be used judiciously.

In general, back corsets or braces should not be used long term as these tend to weaken the abdominal muscles. Instead of contracting these muscles to stabilize the spine, patients tend to push the belly out against the corset, weakening the abdominals. Weight lifting belts are helpful for motorized impact sports like motorcycling and snowmobiling. Skiers can also benefit. In sports like mountain biking where aerobic physical activity is paramount, the belts are contraindicated as these belts will prevent flexion and restrict the diaphragm motion.

Ergonomics

In general, individuals with degenerative disc disease will not like flexion activities. Bending forward loads the painful disc, and many get relief with extension (bending somewhat backward). An exception is cycling, as bending forward is ameliorated by bearing the weight of the upper body on the handlebars.

Sports activities can be modified to reduce stress on the lower back. A classic example is the golf swing. Reducing lumbar rotation and using the shoulders and pelvis more can reduce the stress on the lower discs. With bicycling, shortening the stem and increasing its height can significantly reduce stress. A seat post that is too high can cause pelvic rocking that stresses the discs. Running is more difficult to modify. Wearing shoes that have impact-resistant soles to reduce shock and running on dirt and grass versus a paved course can help. Long hikes can stress the discs and fatigue the core muscles. Hiking poles can reduce impact to the lower back and have an extra benefit of allowing greater upper body conditioning. There is more stress to the spine walking downhill, so poles need to be used.

Skiing can be improved with a more shock-absorbing style and skiing on surfaces that are not as hardpacked to reduce stress. Avoiding moguls is helpful to reduce stress on the spine. A softer ski reduces impact and converts less stress to the lumbar spine. The DIN setting for ski binding release can be reduced. This ensures a softer skiing style as a more aggressive style may overload the spine but cause a premature release, reinforcing a softer style. Swimming is a wonderful form of exercise for severe DDD. It is nonweight bearing, unloads the spine, and is performed in extension, further reducing pressure on the disc.

Occupation can be modified somewhat. Some occupations however require heavy and awkward lifting that degenerative changes in the back may not be able to withstand. However, understanding lifting mechanics may reduce load enough to make the job tolerable. The workplace can be modified to reduce stress on the spine. With standing, such as the occupation of bank teller, a step stool under one foot with alternation of the upward leg can reduce the pressure on one area and make standing more tolerable. Padded floors can reduce standing pressures to relieve back pain.

Sitting positions can be modified to allow more or less lordosis, flexed forward position or somewhat extended. The computer terminal can be raised or lowered depending upon the disorder. A Balans or kneeling-type chair will increase the lumbar lordosis and reduce disc pressure. Simply using an exercise ball for sitting at a desk reduces disc pressure, allows for motion to prevent jelling of the muscles, and contributes to stronger core muscles as the individual must balance while they sit. Just make sure the ball doesn't suddenly deflate or puncture.

Romance and Your Back

There are positions that can aggravate the back when in a romantic mood. Pelvic rocking involves significant extension of the spine, a problem for stenosis, spondylolisthesis, and facet disorders. Standing involves flexion that loads the discs, not the best position for degenerative disc disease. Imagination to discover positions that will not load the spine in a painful manner is the order of the day.

Continued Degenerative Changes

Now for some good news. Father Time was mentioned earlier as being beneficial. Over time, the discs become more degenerative. Yes, this is good news. The more degenerative a disc becomes, the stiffer it is. The stiffer it is, the less motion can occur. Since motion causes pain, as the disc stiffens, the back generates less pain. The problem is, no one can predict how long it will take for the disc to stiffen, and not all discs become stiff with age. Will any individual with chronic disabling back pain improve with time? Many will, but I'm still looking for that crystal ball that will give those answers.

Isolated Disc Resorption (IDR)

This disorder includes all the problems of DDD above with the addition of significant symptom aggregation with impact. For this particular disorder, core strengthening is important, but activity restriction is equally as important. There is no way to help cushion the impact of some activities, and these actions may simply need to be eliminated. Many individuals can still swim, ride a bike (with seat and handlebar adjustment), play golf, and even get into the gym to lift weights with the right body mechanics. Most successful treatments follow the degenerative disc protocol.

Facet Disease

Physical therapy and chiropractic can be effective in treating painful degenerative facets. Facets are loaded when bending backward; therefore, activities that cause extension create pain. The serve or overhead in tennis, swimming, volleyball, and any overhead activity such as painting the ceiling can cause pain. Rotating the pelvis backward flattens out the spine and reduces pressure on the facets. Strengthening the posterior rotators will rotate the pelvis backward. The muscles involved are the abdominals and gluteal muscles as well as the hamstrings. Motion through manipulation may help, but there are times when mobilization is not beneficial. If a degenerative facet correlates with a degenerative spondylolisthesis, mobilization may worsen the slip of the vertebra.

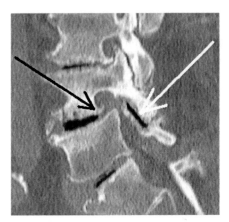

14-5 Degenerative spondylolysthesis—black arrow points
to vertebral slip and white arrow points to worn facet

Sacroiliac Joint Dysfunction

The primary concern here is whether the correct diagnosis has been made. So
many times, the sacroiliac joint is an innocent bystander for referral pain from the
L4-S1 region. If a true sacroiliac disorder exists, treatment includes chiropractic
manipulation, physical therapy modalities, and prolotherapy. In general, injections
of steroid give good diagnosis relief in most cases. In resistant cases, other therapies
can be very helpful. Muscles don't cross this joint, so muscular strengthening is not
very effective. Prolotherapy is the injection of an irritant into the SI joint to stiffen the
joint, kill the pain receptors, and reduce pain (see alternative therapies).

Treatment for Leg Pain

Herniated Disc

In therapies for these radiculopathies, the caregiver needs to strengthen the core
muscles, gently stretch the nerve without aggravating it, and treat any trigger points
that are caused by the nerve compression. Trigger points are discrete tender points
normally found at motor points in muscles that cause local spasm and discomfort.
Continued cardiovascular training during therapy is essential to reduce pain and make
existing pain more tolerable.

The major theme early in the treatment of sciatica is to avoid a flare-up of the
nerve. The therapist has to be careful with the "straight leg raise" maneuver as this
can really irritate the nerve root. Extension and neutral spine exercises are the order
of the day. Only when the nerve is less inflamed and can be gently stretched could leg
flexion exercises be started. If the nerve is stretched too much, especially in the early

stages, a recurrence of the leg pain will occur. The therapist, however, eventually has to start stretching the nerve. Occasionally, the nerve can become irritated even with a gentle stretch. This is truly where the "art" of treatment comes in.

Medications are quite useful for early control of the pain and spasm. If the nerve is really painful, even strong narcotics won't dull the throbbing. This is where an epidural steroid injection is very valuable. After the injection, there can be immediate relief, and the relief can be long standing. Membrane stabilizers can be effective for severe pain early in the disease process.

Resumption of normal activities may take as little as two months to as long as a year. It may take three to six months or longer for certain activity restrictions to be lifted to prevent root pain recurrence.

Foraminal Stenosis and Spinal Stenosis

Both of these stenosis conditions will be aggravated by exercises that cause the back to extend. Walking tends to aggravate the nerve pain unless pelvic tucks are used. That is, to flatten the lower back by tucking the pelvis in (rotating it posteriorly) to increase the room for the nerves. This is done by strengthening the abdominal muscles and the hamstrings. This is the same therapy as the treatment of facet disease.

The same conditions hold for sports and activities. Again, basic core strengthening and endurance training is important. Walking and hiking can be helped with ski poles to allow forward bending, especially with walking downhill. These patients like bicycles, as with the forward bend, there is no leg pain.

Ergonomics of Foraminal Stenosis and Spinal Stenosis

What is interesting is that stenosis patients can normally snow ski all day. As is well-known, a good skier will force his or her weight toward the front of the skis. This requires forward flexion, the maneuver that opens the canal that gives perfect relief for the stenosis patient. These individuals will not, however, like to stand in lift lines. The ski boots force the lower leg into a forward lean. To compensate when standing in the lift line, the patient needs to lean backward, the exact position these patients need to avoid. If you look at skiers while waiting for the lift, they will lean forward on their poles.

The same mechanism is noted with bicycling. Again, a forward lean on the bike opens the spine, and these individuals can bike all day long. In fact, a differential test can be used for these patients without an MRI available. Have the individual pedal on a stationary bike for ten minutes. This should be no problem. Then have them do five minutes on a flat treadmill. They will develop symptoms of claudication. Note that if the treadmill is significantly elevated, they will need to bend forward to keep on it. This could give them enough decompression to negate the test.

"Piriformis Syndrome"

This is a very rare syndrome and as uncommon as the sacroiliac joint causing pain. The first order of business is to be sure the diagnosis is correct. If so, stretching of the muscle is paramount. Local treatment in the form of ultrasound and massage can be helpful.

Isthmic Spondylolisthesis

The first important task if the patient is young is to diagnose the fracture. Any chronic lower back pain in a young individual has to be considered an acute pars fracture unless proven otherwise. The injury is diagnosed by x-rays, a CT scan, and/or a bone scan. Treating the impending fracture as soon as it starts to occur in the young is important as this is the best chance for healing. Treatment starts with reducing the stress on the bone by wearing a flat back brace. Activity restriction takes the load off the bone to allow healing. However, even with the best of treatment, some of these fractures still won't heal.

Even when the fracture is established and won't heal, many of these patients still do not become symptomatic. This is a recurring theme in many spine disorders. The individuals that develop pain develop it much later in life. The defect is uncovered by an episode of lifting or twisting that aggravates the fracture. If patients do develop late pain, it can become a difficult condition to treat short of surgery.

Late treatment is based on pelvis rotation and strength to stiffen the lower back (sounds like the treatment for facet disease and stenosis, doesn't it?). This condition can be helped by "tucking" the pelvis (rotating it posteriorly) to flatten the sacral angle. This positioning reduces the forces on the slip. Again, core strengthening is paramount. Here, the therapist *does not* want to stretch the lower back, but to *reduce motion* of the L5-S1 segment. Motion of the lumbar spine is undesirable as the goal is to stiffen the slip area, not mobilize it. Stretching the hamstrings is a must as these are chronically tight. Stretching muscles next to a structure you don't want to mobilize is a big order to fill. Again, this defines a great therapist.

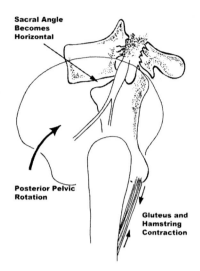

**14-6 Tight hamstrings and reduction
of slip angle of L5**

Degenerative Spondylolisthesis

Patients with symptomatic degenerative spondylolisthesis typically have spinal stenosis. Stenosis patients will unconsciously try to keep their back flat when they walk to keep the canal as open as possible. The only ways to do this are to rotate the pelvis posteriorly and to bend forward. Bending forward while walking wastes too much energy from gluteal muscle contraction. To compensate for this, many will keep their knees bent while walking. This is still very inefficient, but better than the alternative.

Therapy for this condition focuses on core strength (again), but here, posterior pelvic rotation is paramount. Stretching the pelvis while avoiding stretching the slipped vertebra is important. Strengthening and conditioning the abdominals and hamstrings while stretching the psoas muscles keeps the posterior pelvic alignment. If the pelvis won't posteriorly rotate enough, strengthening the quadriceps muscles to allow a bent-knee gait will be helpful.

Scoliosis

For adults, treatment of scoliosis is really the treatment of whatever painful degenerative components occur. Controversial is whether to put scoliosis patients into a stretching or yoga program. On one hand, stretching contracted painful structures will give some relief. On the other hand, scoliosis patients will benefit from avoiding stretching, as avoidance will allow the spine to become stiffer as this will prevent progression of the curve. Progression of the curve can compress a nerve root or allow the deformity to become greater, triggering the need for surgery.

The treatment of children is really a much different discussion. Children's scoliosis is nonpainful. In fact, this is the reason there are scoliosis screenings in school. Kids with a certain degree of curve will increase the size of the curve with growth. The purpose of treatment in young individuals is to reduce the progression of the curve. Brace treatment is designed to prevent the curve from increasing.

Thoracic Hyperkyphosis

An increased thoracic curve needs to be compensated by an increased lumbar lordosis.

This increased lordosis can cause increased strain on the facet joints and premature wear. Standing and loading the spine (lifting and impact) will increase low back pain.

Treating only the lumbar spine will not reduce the stress on the spine. The thoracic spine also needs to be treated. There is no way to really reduce the increased thoracic kyphosis, but strengthening the thoracic extensor muscles and stretching the curve will give some relief. Strengthening the lumbar extensor muscles will help to compensate for the lumbar stress.

Lateral Femoral Cutaneous Nerve Pain

This nerve can be caught under the inguinal ligament. Normally, weight loss if the belly is pendulous will help. Removal of heavy utility belts will reduce stress on the nerve. Injections can be helpful, but occasionally, a surgical release of the nerve needs to be undertaken for severe unrelenting pain.

Lateral Trochanteric Bursitis

This bursal inflammation can be treated by ultrasound, iontophoresis, and stretching of the tensor fascia lata. Local injections of steroid work well but may need to be repeated.

Iliotrochanteric Bursitis

The bursa here is deep to the groin where the tendon of the psoas muscle passes to insert on the lesser trochanter of the hip. The treatment is similar to lateral trochanteric bursitis.

Hamstring Insertional Tendonitis

This disorder is thankfully rare as it is difficult to treat. Stretching of the muscle can help, again is similar to bursitis above. Injections are useful but can occasionally cause avulsion of the tendon from the bone. The surgical repair of this insertional tendonitis can be curative.

How Muscles Recover from Nerve Injury

Muscles have four ways to recover from nerve injury. The first is obviously that the nerve itself recovers quickly, and the signal is reconnected to the brain. We have experienced this phenomenon when we rest our inside elbow on a hard surface. The ulnar nerve is compressed, there is a temporary conduction block, and the outside of the hand "falls asleep." When the pressure is removed, the nerve recovers, and the sensory nerves and muscles work again. The other recoverable cause is that the nerve itself was fully intact, but the surrounding myelin sheath was damaged. Repair of this sheath takes four to twelve weeks before the nerve can conduct again.

The second recovery is with more prolonged compression that actually injures the nerve. If the muscle cell is without nerve input for a period of time, it sends out a chemical signal for help. Any intact motor nerves in the immediate area sprout and send a new branch to the muscle cell. Again, this budding takes ten to sixteen weeks. When the muscle cell is reconnected, the muscle cell can then contract again. On the EMG, this appears as a more coarse contraction. Intact axons can bud up to three to four times. That is, a single nerve can pick up three to four times the number of muscle cells it normally services.

The third is that the nerve, if not too damaged, will regrow down its old pathway and reconnect to the muscle once again. This implies that the pathway for the nerve (the myelin sheath) was not damaged. The nerve will grow down an intact sheath at about one inch per month. An injury to the S1 nerve at the spinal level means that the nerves have to grow down the sheath more than two feet. That means twenty-four months at one inch a month. The problem is that the muscle, without a nerve supply, will become fibrotic, meaning useless, in a period of twelve to eighteen months. Muscles that are eighteen inches or less from the injury, assuming an intact myelin sheath, have a chance of reconnection.

The forth recovery has to do with conditioning. Of course, even if some of the muscle cells are lost because of faulty nerve connections and sprouting does not occur, the remaining muscle cells can hypertrophy (get bigger and stronger) to compensate for the missing cells. This is where therapy can help.

15

Alternative Care For Low Back Pain

Alternate treatments for lower back pain are based sometimes on variations of rational approaches, sometimes on methods that had results but without scientific validation, and occasionally on metaphysical ideas that are not provable on a scientific basis. As far as alternative treatment poses no danger to the patient (other than financial outlay) and there are no dangerous conditions that could be aggravated or made worse with one of these treatments, this is a reasonable way to go.

There is a caveat here. I do tell my patients that if they have no immediate threat and a quartz crystal necklace or a magnet in their belt would give them relief, I would be the first to prescribe it. That being said, there are so many alternative treatments that can be ineffective, so do due diligence.

There is always a new "fad" that pops up every five to ten years that is heavily advertised as a "new CIA finding" or "a secret that doctors don't want you to know." For the most part, this is silly. There are intermittently some newer findings that can be translated into treatment, but this takes years and is generally well-researched. There are no secrets to the treatment of low back pain.

The latest fad is a new form of traction that comes in a very impressive package. It is a large machine with many lights and dials and looks very extraordinary. It is touted as a "NASA" invention (as if NASA is in the business of medical research, especially regarding low back pain). What it really is, and only is, is traction. This had been eliminated sixty years ago as a treatment of low back pain as relatively ineffective. How it arrived now, again, is only through the path of entrepreneurs. Like many "new treatments" before it, the patient must sign up for twenty sessions at considerable cost. This machine may look impressive, but it is just traction. As soon as the patient stands up, gravity "weighs in," and the results of traction are mitigated.

For any new type of treatment, in my opinion, if you don't see relief in five to eight sessions (outside of strengthening and stretching rehabilitation, which takes a while), the treatment will generally not be effective. Do not allow patients to sign up for any program that requires a prolonged series of treatments before "results" can be noted.

Acupuncture

This is the ancient Chinese healing that does not treat an actual medical diagnosis. The basis for acupuncture is to balance meridians that "flow" throughout the body. Needling certain points can allow the "blocked chi" to flow properly and correct whatever ailment this disruption allows to occur.

In my experience, acupuncture can give short-term relief to patients with chronic low back and leg pain, but it is not as effective for long-term care. There are patients with chronic neuropathic pain that don't have good standard medical treatment options. I think acupuncture is a great alternative for these individuals. Unfortunately, it generally only gives short-term relief, but sometimes, this may be one of the only treatment types that is effective for chronic neuropathy.

Trigger Point Injections

Trigger points are discrete areas within a muscle that are extremely tender and palpate as an area of painful chronic muscle contraction. These points have been blamed for the cause of local pain; however, they are normally a result of nerve irritation or chronic muscle contraction. They can occasionally be the direct cause of local pain. A trigger point injection, generally with lidocaine and a steroid, can give temporary and sometimes permanent relief to these painful regions. Many times, however, the systemic steroid effect that occurs twenty-four hours after the injection may be the source for the relief and be misinterpreted as the trigger point injection giving the relief. There is little downside for these injections. They can occasionally cause skin discoloration or ulceration.

Bursal injections are an offshoot of trigger point injections. There is a number of bursa around the hip that can cause pain and mimic a spinal condition. Injection of steroid into the bursa can relieve pain for weeks to months. One condition called iliotrochanteric bursitis is treated very effectively by this injection.

TENS Units (Transcutaneous Electrical Neurostimulation)

Pain pathways can be blocked by flooding the nervous system with stimulation from sensory sources. All of us have done this very maneuver in the past. If you ever injured your arm and then unconsciously briskly rubbed the skin, you found the pain had much decreased from the original injury. What you did was simply flood the sensory system with so many signals you overshadowed the pain fibers.

This simple effect is called the gate theory of pain that was developed in 1965, and it won a Nobel Prize for Melzack and Wall. The useful manifestation of their theory is found in the TENS unit. The TENS unit is a simple battery-powered device that delivers an electrical stimulation via surface electrodes placed on the skin in the area of pain. It obviously doesn't cure the source of pain, but can be quite useful to control pain. These units are normally distributed by chiropractors, physical therapists, and some physicians.

Magnets

There are people who swear by these magnetic devices. I have a friend who sleeps on a magnetic bed and wears magnetic insoles. Needless to say, there is no scientific data to support magnets as a treatment for low back and leg pain. I don't endorse them, but if for whatever reason, magnets give the patient relief, use them. Just don't pay too much for them.

Therapeutic Massage

This is probably familiar to most individuals reading this book. Massage, in its various forms, works on muscles to sooth and relax them. For patients with chronic muscle pain or overuse syndrome (protecting painful structures), it can be very comforting and pain relieving. The benefits are normally temporary, but there are some times that this form of treatment is essential for breaking spasms. Regular massage can give temporary relief but at significant cost, so if it is not therapeutic, it is not warranted.

There are contraindications to massage such as relief of a hypertonic protective muscle contraction. If this muscle is relaxed, the protection given by its hypertonicity will be lost, and back pain after massage will be increased.

Feldenkrais Treatment

This treatment was invented by an Israeli physicist to help with back problems. It involves a series of very small repetitive movements that are designed to "reintegrate" the nervous system. It is effective only in a minority of patients, but it is an alternative choice.

Rolfing

Rolfing is a series of deep tissue massages designed by Ida Rolf for treatment of muscular diseases. It may be as effective as regular deep tissue massage. Don't get contusions by an overenthusiastic rolfer.

Homeopathy

Homeopathy is a form of treatment that was developed in the 1900s by a German scientist. The premise was that certain botanical products or natural elements taken internally would cause a set of discrete symptoms, mimicking the same symptoms as a disease process. By taking the "antidote" to these series of symptoms, the symptoms would be relieved. The antidote was typically made out of the original substance but "strengthened by dilution." That is, the more dilute the substance was made, the stronger the antidote became.

There were some antidotes that were so diluted there was not even one molecule of the original natural substance left in the solution. The theory goes that the solution the original molecule was harbored in "remembered" it and that energy was stored in the solution.

Homeopathy is not too successful in the treatment of back or leg pain. It won't cause a cure of the problem. It however won't cause harm, so there is no downside other than the cost.

Prolotherapy

Prolotherapy is designed to use a caustic injectable substance to promote inflammation and "the healing response." The theory behind prolotherapy is that pain has developed because a ligament or tendon in the back has been stretched. This stretched structure no longer keeps the spine stable, and therefore, aberrant motion and pain has developed. The rationale follows that the way to tighten or strengthen the ligament is to inject it with a slightly damaging substance such as concentrated glycerol or phenol.

The injection causes injury to the tissues and a scar response. The injectable material "promotes healing" with fibroblasts that flow into the injured area and contract when laying down scar tissue. The reaction to this injury is to "tighten up" the area. The areas that are injected may be muscular, tendonous, or ligamentous.

There are some areas of the body that do not respond well to these injections. The exception may be the sacroiliac joint. If truly the pain generator, this joint may become more stable by scarring down the capsule and becoming less mobile. Care has to be taken as if the front of the SI joint is torn and the injected material leaks out, it bathes the sciatic nerve, and damage could result to the nerve.

Injection into the muscles of the lower back is not recommended. Destruction of portions of that muscle group may result, leaving less muscle tissue to cope with daily activities.

16

Chronic Pain, Depression, and the Autonomic Nervous System

Chronic Pain Syndrome

Chronic pain's origin is from tissue damage or from nerve injury. A chronic pain syndrome occurs when the nerve or nerves continue to send pain signals even if the tissue damage has resolved. The nerve signal for unknown reasons continues and *becomes amplified.* Although the literature suggests there may be a personality type associated with this diagnosis, this does not seem to be the typical case. Army rangers and professional athletes develop chronic pain syndromes.

Neuropathic pain can lead to a chronic pain syndrome. The symptoms of neuropathic pain are characterized as burning, tingling, crushing, gnawing, and crawling. Symptoms tend to be worse at night and not generally affected by activity. Allodynia may occur—pain generated by innocuous stimulation of an area occupied by sensitized pressure receptors. It is severe pain provocation on simple stimulation of the skin such as light touch. Eventually, most patients will develop reactive depression as a result of their altered lifestyles.

Depression

Depression can go hand and hand with lower back pain. As early as the seventeenth century, Voltaire stated that "the lower back is at the crossroads where the psyche meets the soma." Patients with painful knees, elbows, and shoulders don't seem to have the same inability to cope with impairment that patients with low back pain have. Low back pain can change a patient's life. Activities that they find pleasurable, ranging from playing tennis and running to sitting at the computer, can become inaccessible because of pain.

The brain reacts to these unpleasant stimuli negatively. Sleeping becomes difficult (insomnia), pleasurable activities are not anticipated (anhedonia), reaction to annoyances becomes out of proportion (irritability), and general fatigue can set in (lethargy).The constellation of these symptoms is called reactive depression. Most or all of these symptoms can be present.

Sensitivity to pain becomes greater with chronic pain and depression. Pain perception is individualized (and may be genetic) with some individuals who can tolerate intense pain and others who cannot tolerate even mild pain. Chronic pain reduces the tolerance to pain of all these individuals. Even strong-willed patients succumb.

As noted in the preceding chapter, the brain can be thought of as having a series of filters that strain out pain from conscious thought. The greater porosity of the filters, the more the pain sensitivity. Chronic pain "increases the pore size" of these filters, making pain more intense and, therefore, less tolerable.

Chronic pain depletes the brain of the chemical transmitter serotonin that is responsible for the general well-being of the brain. A decrease of serotonin causes many nerves to poorly transmit. This condition causes the symptoms of depression.

The SSRIs (selective serotonin reuptake inhibitors) can help make the filter less porous and increase serotonin levels. Serotonin, as a neurotransmitter, is generally absorbed at the nerve ending, reducing its availability. If this reuptake is inhibited, there is more serotonin available to trigger the nerve. This makes the nerves involved more sensitive to serotonin. Serotonins tend to help the "emotional well-being" of the brain, so elimination of this transmitter makes patients more irritable.

There are many SSRIs, and their effects vary. Trial and error is used until the right one is found that has the most beneficial effect.

Chronic Pain Treatment

One of the first keys in chronic pain management is to make sure there is no physical reason a nerve structure is compressed or instability has developed in the spine that can be cured surgically to relieve the pain. If none can be found, then this pain is probably neuropathic (nerve-induced) pain. Reduction of pain through chemical and physical pathways is the next step. Treatment can be reduced to four and possibly five important steps: blocking the pain, making the pain filters stronger, reducing the irritability of the injured nerve, and cardiovascular fitness. The very last step is an implantable device to electrically interference with pain signals.

There are ways to make the brain's filter less porous to reduce the transmission of pain to the brain. One way is through cardiovascular fitness. This increases endogenous endorphins, allows more tolerance of pain in general, and, therefore, "tightens up the filters."

Chronic pain makes these filters much more porous, and chronic pain patients need more narcotic medication to help deal with the pain. Even with some patients who are not depressed, giving the SSRI can help reduce the pain.

Pain medications such as narcotics are helpful in the short term but create more problems in the long term with habituation and addiction. Tachyphylaxis is a phenomenon that occurs when the body develops resistance to continuous use of a medication. The human body regularly develops resistance to narcotic medications.

When tachyphylaxis occurs, the same narcotic dose becomes less effective over time. Nonsteroidal anti-inflammatories such as ibuprofen also block pain signals with much fewer side effects.

Membrane stabilizers are a mainstay for treatment. These slow down nerve sensitivity and can block false signals.

Finally, if there is leg pain greater than low back pain, an electrical stimulator can be surgically implanted on the spinal cord to dilute pain signals.

Autonomic Nervous System Pain (Reflex Sympathetic Dystrophy/ Complex Regional Pain Syndrome)

Reflex sympathetic dystrophy/Complex Regional Pain Syndrome, a chronic pain condition, is an example of damage to the autonomic nervous system.

RSD/CRPS occurs normally after an injury or surgery but can happen even spontaneously. The syndrome is exemplified by severe burning pain and, eventually, trophic changes (loss of skin texture and swelling) in the skin and joints of the involved extremity. Initially (first three months), the patient will have increased circulation, swelling, and color change to the involved extremity associated with the distinct pain. Three to six months later, the swelling will disappear, and the part will be cool with contracted joints but continued pain.

Treatment includes the normal medications for pain, inflammation, and spasm. In addition, the patient normally will get relief with injectable blocks of the sympathetic nerves. The reason why we think the sympathetic nervous system is involved is that blocking these nerves gives the patient relief of pain.

A Side Note to Overstimulation of the Parasympathetic Nervous System—Fainting (Syncope)

The other component of this autonomic system is the parasympathetic component. This is the "housekeeping" part of the system that is important in digestion, reproduction, and elimination. It slows your heart, helps to secrete enzymes for digestion, and controls the function of the sexual organs. When this system is overstimulated, a vasovagal event occurs. Since the parasympathetic nerves temporarily slow down your heart, your brain does not get enough oxygen, and you faint (lose consciousness).

17

Medications, Their Use and Misuse

Medications can be used to modulate many functions in the body. They may actually change the physiology of the damaged tissue or simply block or alter transmission of signals to and from the brain. Medications can be used for pain control, to reduce muscle spasms, reduce inflammation, slow or stop nerve signals, and increase an important but depleted neurotransmitter substance. Most of the time, medications cause a temporary reduction in the pain and discomfort. There are occasions, however, when they can cause a more permanent reduction in the pain.

Medications can be divided in terms of temporary relief, medium term, long term, and possibly curative potential. Temporary uses are such that someone may come in with severe pain, but the course of their problem will be very short term and time limited. Keeping these patients comfortable while the damaged tissue heals requires sometimes large doses of medications on a declining use basis. Once the painful phase is gone, they can comfortably be taken off the medication and start therapy.

Some patients that have severe pain require immediate surgery, and their relief will occur as soon as they wake up from surgery. In this case, strong medications keep them comfortable until surgery can be scheduled.

Medium-term patients are ones that can be made comfortable only after an involved rehab program and activity modification. Sometimes, surgery is an answer for them, but surgery is not contemplated until they have gone through an extensive recovery program. To keep them comfortable, medications are used to allow them to rehab with less pain.

The long-term patients are really "chronic pain" patients. Either their problem will not respond to rehabilitation, they don't want to undergo surgery, or there is no surgery that can help them. These patients are in a special group that requires sometimes lifetime medications. The standard protocols to help pain patients don't apply to them, and their medication programs are very different.

Classifications of Medications

Medications can be classified by their actions. Some stop pain through the opioid pathway, some by stabilizing nerve membranes, and some by reducing the inflammation around the pain receptor.

Narcotics

Narcotics are the most commonly thought of substances for back pain. They are essentially natural or synthetic products derived from the opium poppy. These medications can be very effective to block pain if used appropriately. Narcotics attach to naturally occurring opioid receptors in the brain, spinal cord, and peripheral tissue to block pain signals. These would be wonder drugs except for two significant drawbacks. One is that narcotics attach not only to pain receptors, but also attach to other brain receptors that involve dopamine. This stimulates a euphoric effect—in effect, "a high." This consequence is the reason why these drugs can be so addicting to some individuals. They also act as a depressant that, in larger doses, can cause the brain's drive to breathe to become significantly reduced, sometimes fatally.

The other problem with this category of drugs is the issue of becoming less effective with long-term usage. When opioid receptors in the brain and body are blocked or "full," the brain and body go about creating more receptors. These new receptors again allow the transmission of pain. The new receptors then require more amount of narcotic to cover them. This cycle can continue to go on until the amount of narcotic needed for pain relief becomes excessive. This process is called tachyphylaxis. Eventually, the respiratory drive can be depressed before pain relief can be achieved, leading to death.

Still, with the understanding of these drawbacks, short-term use of narcotics remains the most valuable treatment for acute pain and some types of chronic pain.

Narcotics can be classified in regard to strength, length of effect, and potential side effects. It is important to understand that many narcotic preparations today contain Tylenol and, occasionally, aspirin. Total Tylenol dosage should not exceed 4,000 mg per day. Patients with liver problems should not have Tylenol, and ulcer patients should avoid aspirin. Kidney patients need to reduce the amount of aspirin and Tylenol they use.

The first group is the least potent and most commonly used for mild, chronic pain, and occasionally acute pain. They include Tylenol with Codeine, and Ultracet. All of these have very limited addictive potential but give reasonably good pain relief. Many patients that have chronic problems are on these medications, and they seem to have the least amount of abuse and hypersensitivity potential.

The second group includes Vicodin (hydrocodone) and its derivatives. This is a group that can be used for chronic pain but does have some additional addictive potential. These products are reserved for patients with increased pain and, occasionally, longer-term use.

The third group includes Percocet and its derivatives (oxycodone). These drugs are more effective because of their higher potency and, therefore, more liable to be used by those seeking the "euphoric high." They have more potential for abuse, and sensitivity to them develops more quickly. These are the narcotics most commonly used for postoperative pain control and, occasionally, are useful for longer-term use.

OxyContin is a newer narcotic and is basically timed-release Percocet. Percocet has only a four-hour life span in the body. OxyContin delivers twelve hours of medication without that peak and, therefore, better pain control with not as much euphoria.

The highest potency narcotics are Dilaudid, morphine, and fentanyl as well as methadone. These are used for severe postoperative pain, cancer pain, and, occasionally, chronic pain syndromes. They are used for patients with severe back pain and are not ideal because of their addiction and sensitivity problems.

NSAIDs (NonSteroidal Anti-Inflammatory Drugs)

These medications are of the class similar to aspirin. Aspirin was initially discovered by Native Americans as it comes from the bark of the wintergreen tree; ibuprofen (Motrin) was the first large-scale manufactured NSAID and the first over-the-counter NSAID. These all work by blocking the conversion of arachidonic acid into prostaglandins. Prostaglandins cause inflammation and pain nerves to become sensitized. If this conversion is blocked, inflammation and, therefore, pain will be reduced. Unfortunately, prostaglandins also help to protect the stomach lining from acid, and in some individuals, NSAID usage can cause ulcers.

There are second-generation NSAIDs called COX-2 inhibitors that seem to selectively work on non-stomach-related prostaglandins. These have less chance of causing ulcers. They also seem to have a higher association with cardiac problems. A benefit is that most of them work for twenty-four hours, meaning they are taken once a day. Unfortunately, the price of these drugs is higher than other prescription NSAIDs. Individuals with cardiac issues should not take these medications. The one still on the market is Celebrex.

To be most effective, nonsteroidals generally need to be taken prior to the activity that will cause the pain. If you are planning a day of hiking, take the medication before you head out in the morning. Also remember that Motrin lasts for six hours, so a repeated dose may need to be taken during the activity. Naprosyn (Aleve) does last for twelve hours, so there is less need to repeat doses.

If a patient takes any nonsteroidal on a daily basis, every six months, it is recommended to have a liver profile lab test. There are rare patients that develop liver dysfunction after chronic usage of NSAIDs. If that does happen, most patients improve after stopping the medication.

One major problem with these medications is their capability to reduce the ability of bone to heal after a fracture or even after surgery. Because of this, it is not recommended to use any aspirin or NSAID for three months following a spinal fusion or fracture.

Tylenol (Acetaminophen)

Tylenol is a very good medication. It has the properties as a painkiller and anti-fever drug. It doesn't have the anti-inflammatory effect that NSAIDs do, which is both a benefit and a problem. Tylenol's benefit is that it will not cause stomach problems, which is the major side effect of NSAIDs. Tylenol will not, however, reduce inflammation, which is the major benefit of NSAIDs. The maximum dosage is 4,000 mg per day. This is an important number as many products such as Percocet, Darvocet, and Vicodin all contain Tylenol. An individual may take Tylenol in addition to the above medications at the same time and unknowingly overdose. Since Tylenol does not affect bone healing, patients can use this medication after a spinal fusion.

Muscle Relaxants

This group of medications acts as central depressants (they enter the brain and spinal cord to reduce the input of nerve stimulation to the muscles). Most of these are quite effective to relieve spasm. The price to pay is mild depression of the brain function as these substances also act as a sedative. In fact, one of the indications for these drugs is anxiety. They are good for chronic muscle spasm but have great abuse potential. The prototypical medication in this category is Valium (diazepam). Addiction to Valium is a very difficult condition to treat. This same category of drug can also used as a sleeping aid, important to remember when operating machinery.

There are exceptions to the standard muscle relaxants. One is Flexeril. It is not in the same category as the benzodiazepines of which Valium is a member and has less "tiredness" associated with it. It is an offshoot of the tricyclics that were originally designed for depression. It is not addictive but can make some people "out of sorts" like the effects of Benadryl. Zanaflex (tizanidine) is a medication to reduce muscle spasticity. It has a different action than typical muscle relaxants or Flexeril. Patients with chronic pain, nerve injury causing spasm, and night cramping may benefit. Baclofen (Lioresal) is a medication that was developed for muscle spasm in spinal cord and multiple sclerosis patients but can be effective in patients with cramping and spasm.

Chronic Pain Medications

Membrane Stabilizers

Pain, as we now know, occurs from pain receptors (nociceptors) that are triggered when tissue destruction occurs. This allows us feedback to pull away from a hot surface or to react to an injury (fracture). There are times, however, when the pain nerves themselves are injured and trigger from minimal or even no stimuli. This is called neuropathic pain. Neuropathic pain does not respond well to narcotics or muscle relaxants. What is interesting is that we have found some help from the treatment of epilepsy (seizures).

A seizure focus in the brain is a group of injured neurons that tend to fire without provocation. These nerves are highly sensitive and trigger with minimal or no stimulation. The brain reacts with an amplification response that takes over, and the individual ends up with a seizure. Medications to help this condition stabilize the membranes of these sensitive nerves, so they will be less likely to trigger.

We have found that some of these medications work in the same way with peripheral nerves. The use of these can significantly reduce the pain signals by reducing the pain nerve's ability to propagate the impulse. Of course there can be side effects to this class of medications. One of the most frequent complaints is a feeling of tiredness. In most people, this effect disappears after one to two weeks. In those who have continued lethargy, the medication is reduced and then stopped.

The most common ones are Neurontin, Tegretol, and Topamax and now Lyrica.

Tricyclics

These medications have three benzene rings and, therefore, are called tricyclics. They are older designs of some antidepressants. They have been found to be effective with patients who have sleep disorders and for fibromyalgia. In depression or fibromyalgia, the individual has a problem with getting to sleep, and their sleep cycle is distressed. This, in turn, causes waking-hour irritability. Using these medications can break the sleep cycle disruption and help to make the patient more rested.

Injectables

Obviously, taking an oral medication takes time to get into the system. The medication has to go through the gut and then become absorbed. Also, some of the medication passes right through the digestive tract and doesn't get absorbed. The medication when taken orally becomes distributed throughout the body and does not get concentrated where it is needed.

Giving the same medication through an IV allows a quick, predictable exposure to the medication but again distributes it throughout the body. Injecting it directly into an involved area concentrates the medication where it can be most useful.

Anesthetics

These substances "numb" an area they come in contact with. They temporarily stop the conduction of sensory and, in higher concentrations, motor nerves, so there will be no pain (and sometimes motor) transmission until they "wear off." These medications are useful for minor surgical procedures and to diagnose a pain generator by numbing it temporarily.

Steroids

These naturally occurring substances are the most powerful anti-inflammatories we possess in our arsenal. These medications significantly reduce or stop the nerve pain that occurs from irritation and reduce swelling. This is the one substance that can actually alter the normal course of a back problem. When this is delivered at a higher concentration, it can reduce the inflammation stage (remember, this stage causes the pain) and "cure" the pain. It is not always successful and has some side effects, so it has to be used sparingly.

Narcotics

Local injection of narcotics can be highly successful at reducing pain, especially if injected in the dural sac that surrounds the spinal nerves. They don't have the same euphoric effects as if they were injected into a vein. The problem with them is that they wear off quickly (within four to twenty-four hours) and can cause respiratory depression. They can be constantly delivered by an implantable pain pump.

18

Injections: Diagnostic, Therapeutic, Rhizotomies, Idett, Nucleoplasty, And Discograms

The body is not wired to easily reveal the source of spinal pain. Especially if there is planning for a surgical intervention, knowledge is needed of exactly what structures are involved. Injections however can do so much more than diagnose the pain source. They can be the single most effective treatment for many spinal disorders. This chapter will give you a step-by-step basis for the use of injections.

Diagnostic Injections

To determine the cause of pain, there are many resources that are generally used. The history and physical examination are a great start to reveal the pain source. The MRI and x-ray are the next steps in getting enough information to determine pain generators.

These above tests, however, *do not* always tell us what the source of the pain is. These tests will show us the "geography" of the area. It puts "potential suspects in a lineup," but does not identify the perpetrator. Your doctor, by this point, has a reasonable idea of the various structures that may be causing your pain. The next step is verifying what structure is causing the pain. That role is normally left to the injection.

Does everyone need a diagnostic injection? There would be no reason to do a problem-solving injection if the patient had right leg pain and only one herniated disc pressing on the right nerve root. Here, the diagnosis is obvious, and a diagnostic injection is not needed. However, a therapeutic injection would still be useful to put steroid on the nerve to treat it. The difference between a diagnostic and therapeutic injection will be made clear.

Diagnostic Blocks (Numbing Agents)

An injection can be "diagnostic," "diagnostic and therapeutic," or just "therapeutic." These are code words for the numbing agents like novocaine (diagnostic) and steroid agents (therapeutic). Anesthetizing agents (numbing agents) are the "diagnostic" portion of the injection. If injected around a nerve root membrane, this agent will stop the transmission of sensory impulses from the nerve for about two to four hours. When a particular nerve is suspected of causing the pain, we can inject around the nerve; and if the pain substantially reduces, there is good evidence that this nerve is the cause of the leg pain. Similarly, if a painful facet joint is suspected, the same injection into or around the facet that relieves the pain implicates this joint as the cause of pain.

You have had this nerve block in the past at your dentist's office. Prior to drilling your tooth, your dentist has hopefully and mercifully injected a nerve in the back of your jaw called the inferior alveolar or mandibular nerve with a substance like novocaine. This causes that familiar "dead feeling" in half of your jaw for two to three hours. The dentist has created a temporary conduction block of the nerve. Now, he can happily drill away, and you won't complain (unless you are like me). After two to three hours, your jaw will recover all feeling, but the painful stimulus will have passed.

None of these spinal injections are full nerve blocks. The entire function of the nerve is not blocked. The anesthetic is not injected directly into the nerve itself but placed alongside the nerve membrane to bathe the nerve. This dural membrane filters the anesthetic, so the pain portion of the nerve is blocked, but most of the sensory portions and none of the motor portions of the nerve are blocked (you can still move your leg). However, if a very strong anesthetic is used (4% bupivacaine instead of 0.5% bupivacaine) or inadvertently the medication is injected into the nerve itself, you would get a complete motor block and not be able to move your leg until the anesthesia wore off. Obviously, the correct type and amount of medication needs to be used.

Corticosteroids (Therapeutic Blocks)

The "therapeutic" portion of the injection is a corticosteroid. These are not the steroids that Arnold Schwarzenegger has used (anabolic steroids—a totally different medication). Corticosteroids are naturally occurring substances in the body produced by the adrenal glands. These medications are the most powerful anti-inflammatory the body produces, and physicians have it in concentrated form in the drug arsenal.

Normally, the inflammatory response is important to healing. When you cut yourself, the body goes through a cascade of steps to cause the injured area to heal. A blood clot forms. Blood vessels grow into this clot to bring growth factors to heal. White blood cells diffuse into the area to clean up all the dead and injured cells and tissue. Scar tissue grows into the area to repair the defect. All this orchestrated commotion goes into healing.

The problem is that this healing mechanism can be injurious to nerves. Nerves are very sensitive to their chemical environment and are also sensitive to pressure. When you rest your elbow on the counter and your hand "falls asleep," you have compressed the ulnar nerve at the elbow, and it stops conducting. A herniated disc or bony narrowing of the spinal canal causes two problems: chemical inflammation and mechanical compression.

Mechanical compression (the volume of the herniation or the bone spur) causes direct pressure on the nerve root. This physically prevents the nerve from functioning by deforming the nerve and blocking the transport of nutrients through the cell, slowing the nerve membrane blood circulation and causing the nerve membrane to malfunction.

The disc herniation or spur also causes chemical inflammation because of the nature of the herniation material and the reaction to the spur. Inflammation causes a number of problems. It causes the nerve cell membrane to become more porous. This exposes the nerve to more local contaminants to make it malfunction. White blood cells are called into the area (a process called diapedesis) and release their caustic contents that injure the nerve membrane.

Steroids have many effects that counteract the inflammatory forces that these spinal nerves are subjected to. Steroids hamper the (migration) diapedesis of white blood cells into the nerve area so these cells don't release their caustic contents. Steroids also reduce swelling so the pressure on the nerve itself is reduced. Finally, steroids reduce the pore size of the membrane of the nerve root to make it less exposed to a harmful environment. Nerves "love" this medication because all of steroids' actions counteract the problems caused by the herniation or compression. If it seems to be the perfect medication to treat these problems, that is because it is. However, there are some potential side effects that are rare but need to be discussed.

Many patients are concerned about side effects they have heard about regarding steroid use. Most of these effects are noted when these drugs are taken orally for certain diseases like rheumatoid arthritis. This means that day in, day out, the body has a much higher systemic dose of steroids than it is designed to tolerate. The results of this constant exposure can be debilitating.

An injection of steroid in the spinal area is a one-time dose with the majority going right to the area it is needed. Contrary to belief, this injection will not, by itself, cause osteoporosis. There is a very rare portion of patients who can get avascular necrosis (death of the bone) of a joint such as the hip joint. This can cause arthritis in the joint. A rare patient can get a cushingoid response (their face will swell up temporarily) or gain some water. The more common (but still rare) responses are stomach upset and a "wired" feeling, giving the patient more energy but making them get less sleep. These effects disappear when the medication stops. Steroids can upset the sugar balance in a diabetic, and this needs to be compensated for through more insulin usage.

The use of injectable steroids can be up to three injections every six months. I have some patients that are going on their twelfth year of steroid injections without deleterious effects. Many patients with long-term injectable steroid use, however, do develop resistance. They note the steroids are less effective over time.

Nerve Block Techniques and the Pain Diary

If the physician that is treating you wants to be certain that a particular nerve root is causing pain, he will have the nerve temporarily numbed through a procedure called an SNRB (selective nerve root block). This injection has to be done by an experienced physician as if some numbing substance leaks beyond the nerve to be tested and other nerves are inadvertently also numbed, this may give a false sense of relief (called a false positive test).

Typically, your physician will ask you to aggravate this pain prior to the injection by doing the activity that reproduces the pain (walking, climbing stairs, prolonged sitting, and bending). Obviously, you have to be experiencing the typical pain you normally have prior to the test. You can't numb something that doesn't hurt in the first place.

The exception to this is if your pain is associated with an activity that can be done immediately posttest, like walking or climbing stairs. Directly after the test, do that painful activity to determine if the pain has been relieved. Remember, there is only a two-to-three-hour golden window to discover if the pain improves. After that, the medication wears off, and the diagnostic portion of the test is lost.

The physician ordering the test will ask you to fill out a pain diary so you can accurately record your findings before, at the time of the test, and after the numbing medication wears off.

Some people are nervous about the injection and require sedation while receiving it. Sedation prior to the injection is acceptable only as long as it is a short-acting medication (lasting fifteen to thirty minutes). If you are given a longer-term sedative and you are "drugged up" until after the numbing agent wears off, you will be incapable of determining the effect of numbing the nerve, and the test will be useless. Also, if you are on a strong painkiller, you should be off it generally four to twelve hours prior to the injection.

Types of Injections (Diagnostic and Therapeutic)

Caudal epidurals are the simplest type of intraspinal injection. This injection cannot be used diagnostically as it covers too broad an area to be useful. There is generally no need for an x-ray or fluoroscopy. These are injected by simply palpating the hole (sacral hiatus) at the base of the tailbone (sacrum) and can be done in the office. One of the problems with this injection is that it takes a large amount of fluid (20-30 cc) to reach the area inflamed and cannot always reliably be used to deliver medication to the area. In my opinion, these are generally outdated injections and should only be used in rural areas that don't have fluoroscopy (real-time x-ray) and, only then, by an experienced physician for lower low back problem areas (L4-S1).

Selective nerve root blocks are just as they imply. Only one nerve root is selected for injection, and the spinal canal (where there are many more nerves) is not injected. This test is valuable to identify if a specific nerve is causing pain. These are used for diagnostic as well as therapeutic (treatment) purposes.

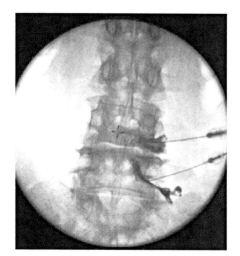

18-1 Selective nerve root block with dye tracing nerve root path

Epidural steroid injections (ESIs) are one of the most common forms of injections. This puts the medication directly into the spinal canal where it bathes the disc and nerves. It is normally very effective for pain relief, but its diagnostic value is less important. It is considered a "shotgun" approach. Its one diagnostic value is for central stenosis. An injection in the area of central stenosis should give three hours relief of the stenosis symptoms. If there are technical problems with the posterior approach, this injection can be put in the canal through the nerve foramen with the same effect. In this case, it is called a **transforaminal epidural steroid injection (TFESI)**.

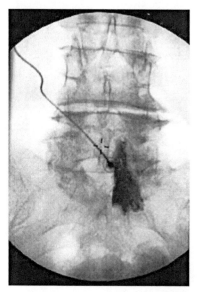

18-2 AP X-ray of epidural steroid injection with dye in canal

Sacroiliac Blocks

The sacroiliac joint only rarely causes pain. If it is suspected, this diagnostic block can be useful. The joint is a very complex one. Portions of it are diarthrodial. That is, it is a normal joint with a joint space and cartilage. However, the inferior one-third of it is just heavy fibrous tissue, and there is no place to easily put a needle to inject numbing material. The front of the joint also lies right next to the sciatic nerve, and if there is a tear in the front of the joint, the nerve may also be numbed. Dye should be introduced into the joint first to make sure it does not leak out in front. This injection is normally diagnostic and therapeutic.

Facet Blocks

Facet injections are of two different types. One can inject medication directly into the facet capsule. This is designed to numb the facet, but in doing so, the capsule is distended. Occasionally, there can be increased pain with this injection (a false negative) as the swollen capsule is stretched. Also, if there is a tear of the capsule and the anesthetic leaks onto the nearby nerve root, a false reduction of pain may be noted (false positive test). Obviously this would give a wrong answer to the question of the facet being a pain generator.

The other technique is to inject the two or three small nerves that supply pain fibers to the facet. These are called the median branches, and there are two to three of them to each facet. The injection is called a medial branch block and is a good way to temporarily deaden these nerves. The caution here is that if the medication leaks down to the central nerve or the disc fibers, the test will again give false relief (a false positive.) This may relieve the pain by deadening the central nerve or disc fibers that is misguidedly interpreted as the facet causing the pain.

If these injections are repeated with the same excellent results (a substantial portion of pain is relieved), then this provides reasonable proof that the structure is the pain generator. Interventional planning can be performed to reduce the pain from this generator (rhizotomy).

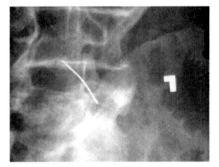

18-3 Fluoroscopy of facet block—needle is in facet joint

Rhizotomy (Dorsal Root Neurolysis)

If the facet is diagnosed as the actual pain generator, a procedure can be done that destroys only the nerve supply to the joint without damaging any other structures. It is called a dorsal facet rhizotomy. In this technique, a small needle is put through the skin onto the sensory nerve, and the needle tip then heats up, cauterizing the nerve in the process. This is done normally under sedation, so the patient doesn't feel any pain. The success rate is close to 70 % with the appropriate diagnosis and technique, but it may need to be repeated as these sensory nerves do grow back under some circumstances.

IDETT

This stands for intradiscal electrothermal therapy. Essentially, a small wire is fed into the disc through a needle. The end of this wire circles around and lies against the annulus (donut) of the disc. The wire is heated up and cauterizes the inside of the disc. The purpose of this is to melt the collagen to "heal" the holes in the disc and to burn any nerve endings that might be painful (similar to the rhizotomy for facets). The initial reports of this technique were quite promising, but the current results have been dismal. Patients who have had this done have not had much or any relief.

Nucleoplasty and Chymopapain

These two processes are designed to reduce the pressure on the annulus by removing some of the nucleus. It would be similar to letting some of the air out of a tire. Chymopapain was the first procedure to be tried. The injected material is made from papaya enzyme and was highly successful in removing most of the nucleus. One problem was that if there was a large through and through tear of the disc, some of the material would leak out through this tear into the canal, causing damage to the spinal nerves (called transverse myelitis). This technique was generally abandoned.

Nucleoplasty is a technique where a larger bore needle is inserted into the disc to remove some of the nucleus. It can be done with laser, mechanical technique, or ultrasonic technique. No matter what the technique, some of the internal nucleus is removed. It may reduce some pressure on the pain nerve fibers for lower back pain. It has value in treating a painful nerve root where the pain from the nerve root is from chemical irritation through a tear in the annulus and not from mechanical compression from a herniation. Results are fair, and the technique has mixed results.

Discograms—Provocation Testing

As you can see, you can numb a structure to see if it gives pain relief. There are some structures that this technique does not work for, most notably the disc. Disc pain will not be relieved by numbing it so a block will not work. This is because the pain nerves are sequestered—they cannot all be reached by injecting the numbing medication.

A technique has been designed to be reasonably reliable to tell us if the disc is causing pain. This test is called a discogram. With it, a needle is placed into the disc in question, and x-ray dye with antibiotic is injected. The inside of the disc (the nucleus) is pressurized. Increasing the pressure inside the nucleus then increases the pressure on the outer rings of the annulus. Increased annular stress will activate the pain receptors in the annulus and, if the disc is the pain generator, should recreate the typical lower back pain. This is called a provocative test, i.e., you provoke the disc with pressure.

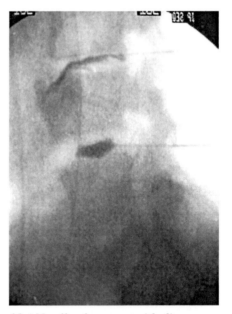

18-4 Needle placement with discogram

Discograms should be done in multiples and blinded. That is, at least two discs should be tested, and one should be a normal-looking disc based upon MRI. The patient should not be informed what disc is being tested (a blinded study). A valid discogram should include a nonpainful disc. A normal nonpainful disc may create a "pressure sensation" but should not be overtly painful. If the discographer inadvertently injects into the annulus, even a normal disc will cause pain, so technique is very important. If normal discs are injected properly and are still painful, the discs themselves may not be pain generators, and the problem may be a "pain-processing problem" in the central nervous system.

Discograms can be "titrated." This means that the discographer will attempt to distinguish between the pain levels of different discs. Even with this technique, a normal disc should be included to rule out pain-processing issues.

The Technique of Discography

The suspected discs and at least one normal disc are interrogated. Under deep sedation, under meticulous sterile conditions, needles are placed into the discs in question. The patient is awoken with the needles already in the discs. Needles already in the discs are not painful. Just as many of you have had an IV, and after the IV catheter is in, you don't feel it. The patient has to be alert and responsive to be able to report how they feel when the discs are pressurized. The discs are injected with a water-soluble x-ray dye mixed with antibiotics. This dye will show up on x-ray as a dark fluid.

The technique is extremely important. First, the needle has to be in the center of the disc. If it is in the edge of the disc or annulus, there will be pain generated by injection, regardless of whether the disc itself has caused pain or not. Second, the patient cannot be sedated once the injection begins. Any significant sedation and the patient won't be able to describe what he or she feels. Third is that some lower discs are hard to put a needle into, and occasionally, information may not be able to be obtained. The greater the skill of the discographer, the less occasions this will occur.

Discs are pain rated as P0, P1, and P2. P0 is no pain with injection (mild pressure is not considered pain). P1 is back or leg pain with injection but not noted by the patient to be the typical pain they normally experience. This pain is called nonconcordant. P2 is the typical and exact back pain the patient normally experiences. The pain is rated by the typical VAS (visual analog scale).

The disc appearance is also noted. A normal disc will hold the dye in its center and will not diffuse into the annulus that would indicate a tear of the disc. A torn disc will have dye leak into the annulus and may allow the dye to leak out the front or the back of the disc.

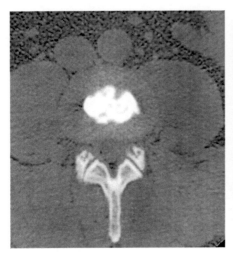 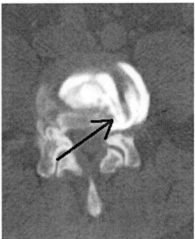

18-5A CT scan of discogram
of normal disc

18-5B CT scan of discogram
of torn disc—arrow points to
tear of back wall of annulus

A very degenerative disc will occasionally have so many tears in it that it will not pressurize, and the dye will flow out as quickly as it is injected. In this case, even if the disc is the pain generator, it will not pressurize and, therefore, will not create pain. This is a false negative test (the disc is the pain generator but will not test positive because of the extensive tears).

This test needs to be blinded. That is, the patient should not have a clue as to what disc is being tested. Two responses would create doubts with the results of this test, making it a nonvalid test. These include pain produced in a normally appearing disc (no tears) and nontypical pain (not the day-to-day pain) from a degenerative disc. The information from this can be used to possibly plan surgery or even to exclude surgery from future planning.

Patients may have pain-processing issues that are mediated by the central nervous system and not mechanical pain from a painful disc. A good test for this is the painful but normal disc upon discogram testing. In my opinion, with some exceptions, this would rule out a patient for a fusion procedure. Done properly, the discogram is a valuable tool to help diagnose a patient if they might need surgery and a valuable tool to help rule out a patient for surgery.

19

Surgical Treatment

Yes, I've heard it all. "Never get back surgery as you'll never be the same." "I don't know anyone who has gotten better from surgery." "All my friends who have had back surgery are worse now." The memories of poor results continue to exist, even results from thirty years ago. Times and knowledge have obviously changed dramatically since then. The current success rate for surgery should be up to 95% in many cases. This is because of our much greater understanding of back problems and what surgery will and won't do. The technical ability of surgeons has improved dramatically, and the tools we have to work with are significantly better. Our ability to diagnose problems is light years better than before the MRI and advanced CT scanners. The further understanding of anatomy and pathology has improved our comprehension. The implants we use have had years for refinements to occur.

Before considering surgery, there are questions to be asked. What type of surgery do I need? Am I a good candidate for the proposed surgery? What are the goals, and what can I expect of the surgery? What is the success rate? How long does it take to recover? What does the recovery entail? What are my responsibilities for surgical success? All are great questions, and all should be asked and answered before contemplating surgery.

Why does surgery work? There are specific disorders that occur with age, trauma, and genetics. These disorders are compressive, mechanical, and alignment associated. This means leg pain from nerve root compression, pain from motion of a degenerative disc, and a collapsing spine that makes the body work harder to stay upright.

Essentially, as there are three types of disorders that can occur, the spine can be modified three different ways surgically to oppose these disorders. The spine can be decompressed (take pressure off a nerve or group of nerves), a segment can be fused because of instability or painful degeneration, and the spine can be realigned due to segmental collapse or scoliosis. Another alternative, disc replacement can also be considered.

When is surgery needed? With some exceptions, the best way I can answer it is with a quote from the famous Supreme Court justice William Potter Stuart. He was once asked if he could define "pornography." He said, "I can't define it, but I know it when I see it." This is the perfect quote for surgery. Most of the time, no one can tell you when you need surgery. You "will know it when you see it." A physician can discuss with patients the description of surgery, the success rate, the potential complications, what to expect, and what not to expect. The patient has to weigh the benefits, success rate versus the risks, recovery, and expectations that they bring. Ultimately, the patient will have to decide if surgery is right for them.

Types of Surgery

Decompression for a Herniated Disc (HNP)

In this disorder, the disc has torn through the outside annulus (the plies of the tire), and the nucleus (jelly) has pushed out. This jelly aggravates the nerve, and the nerve is inflamed and compressed. The compression causes buttocks and leg pain. The symptoms are typical: leg pain, numbness, and a "pins and needles" sensation down the leg. The leg may be weak because the nerve can't transmit the signal for the muscle to respond.

Is surgery required, and if so, when? As noted before, most patients with a herniation can be treated conservatively. This means that with an appropriate course of therapy, medications, injections, and activity restrictions, about 70% of patients will improve enough to calm down most symptoms and return to normal activity. This does however take time. Normally about three months, give or take, to be back to a minimal of "seminormal." Some patients take up to a year, and others never fully recover. The patients who have continued or intolerable pain will eventually need to have surgery. It is up to the patient to decide how much pain is enough. There are some who, after an epidural injection, do just fine and others that have so much pain they need to be admitted to the hospital for intravenous pain medications.

Are there patients that have a pressing need for surgery? The answer is somewhat controversial, but yes. These patients are the group that exhibit muscle weakness. This is not pain inhibition weakness but true neurological weakness. This failing indicates significant compression of the nerve. It takes a larger amount of pressure to make the motor portion of the nerve stop working. The muscles involved may have permanent weakness if there is motor nerve involvement, so in my opinion, surgery should be much sooner than later.

There are some arguments against immediate surgery. Without surgery, it is estimated approximately 50% of the patients will recover good useful motor strength. But that begs the question, what happens to the other 50%? These patients obviously don't recover full or useful motor strength.

Can quick surgery help the chance of recovery? The answer is yes, but it is not 100%. Probably 70-80% of patients will recover useful strength with surgery. Is the extra 20-30% chance of recovery worth the surgery? In most cases, I believe the answer is yes, but other physicians would disagree. The rare exception to avoid surgery with motor weakness is if the patient would be under greater risk from the surgery than the resultant functional deficit from weakness.

This surgery can be performed one of three ways: discectomy, microdiscectomy, or endoscopic discectomy. The goal is simply to remove the offending fragment from the nerve root. The term "discectomy" is really a misnomer as it means "removal of the disc," and the entire disc is never removed. The correct term would be "discotomy," as it really means partial removal of the disc. Results should be about the 95% range for success rate. The reason why it can't be 100% is that it is easy to remove the offending fragment from the nerve root, but the nerve needs to recover. That is up to Mother Nature.

The surgery can be done with the naked eye or with loops that magnify two to three times. This is called a discectomy. This normally necessitates a slightly longer incision, but the results should be quite good. *Microdiscectomy* is the same surgery but done under a microscope. This may have some advantages such as better lighting, a smaller incision, and the assistant looking at the same view as the surgeon. An *endoscopic discectomy* is done with an endoscope, a little TV camera at the end of a probe. These are similar to the ones commonly used for knee arthroscopy. The incision can be the same size as a microdisc surgery or possibly smaller.

Again, in the right hands, all of the above should work well for surgery, and the results should be about 95% success.

Technique—Posterolateral Discectomy

The technique is quite simple. The patient is placed in something like a rounded back or kneeling position. This is done to flatten the spine and "open up" the area between the bony lamina. This reduces the amount of bone that needs to be removed to access the canal that the nerve resides. It also reduces the pressure of small veins found in the canal to reduce bleeding during surgery as the belly "hangs." After the back is prepped (sterilized), markings are made on the skin, and one or two needles are placed in the muscles alongside the spinal column. An x-ray is taken, and the levels are identified.

A small incision (one-half to one inch) is made over the spine, and the fascia is exposed. The fascia is a thin flat "ligament" that the back muscles attach to. This is incised, and a small muscle (the multifidi) is moved over to expose the space between the lamina. Depending upon the level, a small amount of bone may be removed from the inferior lamina to make enough room to safely get into the canal. Performed appropriately, there won't be any side effects from this removal.

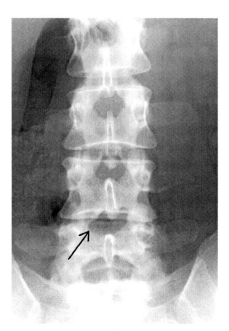

19-1 X-ray of microdisc—arrow points to minimal bone removal

The structure that needs to be removed to get access to the canal is the ligamentum flavum. This is a vestigial structure that lines the back of the spinal canal. Removing it causes no harm. Once removed, the canal is exposed. The compressed nerve will normally be pushed up to the back of the canal as the disc herniation displaces it underneath. It is a simple matter to gently roll the nerve to the inside, expose the herniation, and remove it. The surgeon then finds the tear in the back wall of the disc (the exit point for the herniation). Using a small "grabber" tool, the surgeon reaches into the disc, and any loose fragments are removed to prevent future herniations.

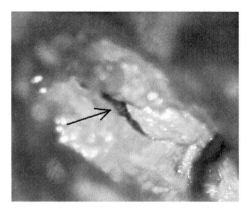

19-2 Picture through microscope of annular tear—
arrow Nerve is being retracted

A small probe is used to sweep under the nerve to make sure there are no further fragments that are not visible (there is a great deal of "feel" to spine surgery). The disc is irrigated to make sure no loose fragments are left. A Valsalva maneuver (done by the anesthesiologist) is used to make sure there is no leak out of the lining of the nerve. After that, some surgeons put a small amount of steroid on the nerve to reduce swelling. The muscles are reattached, and the incision is closed. A drain to remove oozing blood is occasionally used.

Technique—Far Lateral Discectomy

There is a herniation that does not occur within the canal but on the outside side of it. This herniation still compresses the nerve, but to get to it, the access point is different. A far lateral approach requires the same patient position as the standard discectomy with all its inherent benefits. The incision is made off center, and here, the back muscles are separated to gain access to the outside of the disc. Again, the offending fragments are removed, and the incision is closed.

Recovery and Rehabilitation

The patient wakes up in the recovery room normally unaware that surgery has occurred. This is because of preoperative medications that actually prevent memory from storing any experience that occurs prior to or during surgery. Depending on the situation, some patients may go home the same day, but most go home after a twenty-three-hour stay. Just about everyone is up and walking the day of surgery.

The recovery should be quick and reasonably easy. For nearly all patients, the leg pain should be significantly improved. There will be some incisional soreness, but this is usually very mild. After a short period of activity restriction (no bungee jumping or pole-vaulting), the physical therapist will see the patient for a short course of strengthening and education. Most people will be at 90% recovery in three to four weeks and can slowly get back to golfing, skiing, biking, and many other activities.

Problems That Can Occur Postoperatively

Occasionally, after surgery, when the pressure is taken off it, the nerve root can swell, and some discomfort can return for a short period. This normally dissipates over a few weeks with medication

One of the problems with a herniated disc is recurrence rates. The original tear in the disc that allowed the jelly to squeeze out never fully heals (remember the disc has little to no blood supply). That same unhealed hole can still extrude another herniation fragment in the future. This could occur in two days or ten years. The chances of that happening are one in twenty or about 5%. This recurrence rate generally holds even if you don't have surgery. Another way to look at it is the odds are nineteen in twenty that you will never have another problem—not bad odds indeed.

You might reason that the disc should be emptied of all of its contents at the time of surgery to prevent further herniations. A good thought, but that would lead to a lack of shock absorption, possible progressive low back pain, and fragmentation of the cartilage end plates. These end plates, when they fragment, could lead to further loose fragments and then herniations and actually be much more painful. They are hard-edged as compared to the soft original nuclear fragments.

Why can't we just stitch or glue the hole in the disc? Remember, the disc has no blood supply, so suturing the hole won't help as it won't heal. Also, the torn fibers retract. Just like a broken guitar string, they are under tension and won't reapproximate when they tear. There have been past attempts to repair these tears, all with poor results.

Well, then you ask, why don't you just fuse this segment? Fusion is a much more complex surgery and has a much longer recovery. It is saved for patients with significant *back* pain that doesn't respond well to conservative measures or for discs that constantly spit out fragments that can reinjure the nerve.

So the best technique for relief of leg and buttocks pain is to remove the offending fragment off the nerve root and any loose fragments within the disc. The best motto for spine surgery is to do the smallest surgery for the maximum benefit.

Central Decompression (Laminectomy and Its Variants)

The spine over time in most people becomes degenerative. There is no way currently to stop this process. When degeneration occurs, bone spurs form. Remember enthesopathy? These spurs can grow into and narrow the central canal. "Central stenosis" is the term for the narrowing of this passageway. This stenosis causes undue pressure on the central group of nerves, and symptoms of "neurogenic claudication" occur (see chapter 23). Again, if all conservative measures fail and the symptoms become intolerable, surgery is warranted.

The procedure of choice is a laminectomy or variant of such. Again, terminology is not fully accurate as many times the entire lamina is not removed (the definition of lamin**ectomy**). Bilateral hemilaminectomy, bilateral microdecompression, or a horizontal laminotomy (removing a portion of the lamina to make more room) is often used. This procedure opens the central canal and makes room for the nerves.

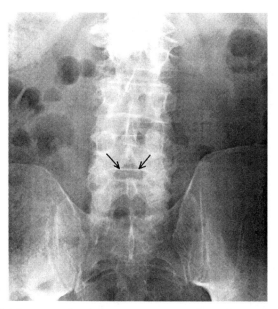

19-3 L4-5 post op laminotomy—arrows point to bone removal

A full laminectomy is the procedure done by removing the entire lamina. This has some advantages as it gives excellent access to the areas of narrowing without obstruction. The surgeon can work from the opposite side of the table, and the ability to angulate the decompressive tools allows better access and more complete decompression along with the ability to get to difficult-to-reach places with less stress on the neurological structures.

Using a laminectomy, the entire canal can be opened, and there are no areas that cannot be visualized or accessed to ensure complete decompression. Other techniques that are less invasive are depended upon more by the "feel" of the surgeon and not visualization.

Using a laminectomy, more material is removed including supra and intraspinous ligaments that could lead (at least theoretically) to greater chance of instability. Therefore, this procedure should not be done by itself if there is any significant evidence of instability (slip with increased motion on flexion/extension x-rays) or impending instability. A stable degenerative disc or a patient who has low demand (elderly or nonathletic, nonheavy work) can have this procedure, and it is considered the "gold standard" for central decompression.

Fusion

The purpose of fusion is to cause two or more bones of the spine (the vertebra) to grow into one. This stops the motion of the disc or facet that causes pain. It is done for four reasons: a painful disc that has failed to be managed any other way, instability (painful abnormal vertebral motion), to open up a collapsed foramen compressing a nerve, and for scoliosis/kyphosis (malalignment of the spine).

The key to successful fusion is to alter the spine into creating a simulated fracture environment. When the bones of the spine are stripped of their attachments and "bone skin" (periosteum), it simulates a broken bone and the reaction to heal. If bone graft or a simulated substance is placed in between the stripped bony structures, the bone will "heal" into its neighbor, creating a fusion.

Rods and Screws (Motion Elimination)

Bone cells need a special environment to grow. These special cells lay down a protein backbone. Other cells follow that, then cause crystallized calcium to be deposited. These crystals finally join together and attach to the existing bone surfaces, eventually resulting in two bony surfaces turning into one solid piece of bone. This is the way any natural break in a bone heals.

Motion is one of the problems that cause these bone cells to break down. Movement will destroy the attempt of the bone cells to heal into its neighbor. We learned this from management of leg fractures. Prior to surgical management of most tibia fractures, orthopaedists would put these fractures in a long leg cast. This was easy, but the cast still allowed some motion at the fracture site, and many of these breaks did not heal. Other times, the healing took over a year, causing debilitation of the patient.

This brings up an interesting historical point. After World War II, some of our soldiers coming back from Germany who were prisoners of war were released. The Department of Defense found that the rare prisoners had steel pins placed in their legs. Initially, the Defense Department thought this was some kind of torture technique. It turns out that the Germans were ahead of us in fracture management. These servicemen had fractured legs, and the rigidity of these rods helped the leg fracture to heal faster and more completely.

Our orthopaedists took quick note and started putting similar rods into long bone fractures to make them more rigid. The healing rate significantly improved. We found that making the fracture more rigid promoted the bone cells to heal.

The same concept is utilized with a fusion of two vertebrae. Pedicle screws and rods are used to connect the vertebra to make them rigid. This improves the chances of fusion and allows the surgeon to place the vertebrae in correct alignment and lock them into place. It also makes the rehabilitation quicker as the surgical area is rigid right from the start.

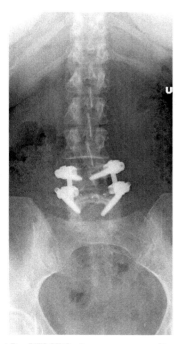

19-4 X-ray AP of TLIF fusion—note small metallic dots
in the disc space from the spacer cage

Fusion Techniques

There are two areas of the vertebra that a fusion can be performed, the posterolateral aspect (facets, lamina, and transverse processes) and the anterior (discs/vertebral bodies). There are certain reasons why one can be chosen over another or both done together. Screw and rods are normally used to augment the fusion.

Posterolateral Fusion

The most common fusion is posterolateral. This fusion joins the facets and transverse processes together. Screws and rods are used to mechanically join the vertebrae. It is the easiest fusion to perform technically and has the least amount of nerve manipulation needed. There is a very reasonable fusion success rate of greater than 90%. As long as the patient has a low physical demand, the satisfaction rate is very high. Why low demand? This technique does allow some minimal motion as it does not fuse the front bodies where the disc is located. With a high-demand patient, this micromotion may be somewhat uncomfortable.

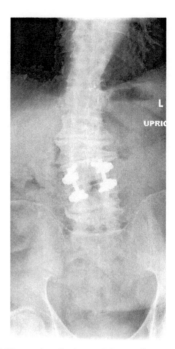

19-5 Posterior fusion without the cage—
this is called a posterolateral fusion

The ALIF

A fusion can be done just from the front of the spine. This procedure is called an ALIF or anterior lumbar interbody fusion. Obviously, the incision needs to go through the belly to get there. Opening the belly and moving the structures is a more challenging technique. There is, however, wonderful exposure of the disc, so the quality of preparation for the bed of fusion is excellent. Bone graft can be packed well into the disc, and a support structure to hold the disc space open can be placed easily. Holding the vertebrae rigidly is somewhat more of a technical problem. This is because you can't easily get mechanical support such as a screw and rod complex to hold the two vertebrae together to stop the motion of the segment. The motion of the segment before the bone grows across may rarely prevent fusion.

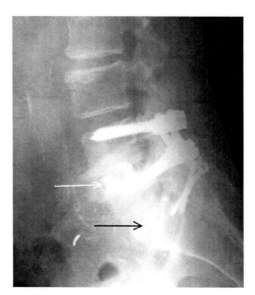

19-6 ALIF fusion along with pedicle screws—white arrow points
to new ALIF and black arrow points to past ALIF

The "360"

There are times that a fusion procedure can be done with both surgery from the
front and the back at one setting. This is called a 360 fusion as the surgery is done in
a 360-degree plane (front and back). This makes the time of surgery somewhat longer
as there are two approaches to be made. When this procedure is warranted, the success
rate for fusion is very high.

The TLIF

One procedure called a TLIF (transforaminal lumbar interbody fusion) can
perform this "360" fusion of both the disc space and the posterolateral structures
from an approach just in the back. There is an area of the disc where there is natural
space between the two nerve roots. This area has enough room to remove most of the
degenerative disc and place in a spacer and fusion bone. The procedure is technically
more challenging but has the advantage of creating a fusion in an area that is normally
approached only from the front, saving an invasive belly surgery. The standard
posterolateral fusion is performed at the same time with pedicle screws.

This is called a TLIF because on one side, the facets need to be removed to allow the
angulation necessary to clean out the entire disc and place fusion bone across it. A disadvantage
of this technique is that the surgeon is working around the nerve roots that can occasionally be
quite sensitive to disturbances. This makes the procedure more meticulous and demanding.
There can occasionally be nerve irritation that occurs from the procedure.

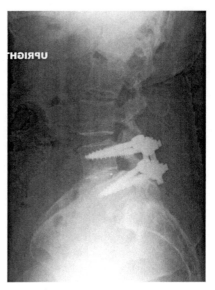

19-7 TLIF fusion lateral X-ray

The advantage to the procedure is that the bony surfaces that are exposed by the facet sacrifice (the discal end plates) have a much greater surface area and ability to fuse. Also, for instability pain, the pain generator itself (the disc) is removed. Another advantage of a TLIF is the opening of the foramen. By distracting the two vertebral end plates, the hole the nerve lives in (foramen) is enlarged. Any nerve root caught by bone spur in the foramen is freed. Bone taken from the removed facet can be used for fusion, obviating the need for a bone graft from the pelvis.

Breakdown Above and Below a Fusion

A long fusion can theoretically put increased stress on the disc above or below the fusion. A question is, can this increased stress create overload pressure and break down the next disc in line? There is no question that in long fusions for scoliosis, leaving just one or two discs open below will cause breakdown of these discs prematurely. In general, with an isolated fusion of L5-S1, the chance to see problems develop above is not high. A fusion from L4-S1 (two levels) can increase the stress of the next disc up, and patient's activity level has to be somewhat reduced after this type of fusion. Occasionally, a three-level fusion has to be performed for fracture, scoliosis or instability, and, rarely, low back pain. Normally these patients with scoliosis or instability have significantly reduced active lifestyles but still tend to do well with these surgeries.

It seems that genetics plays a significant role in disc breakdown. If the disc at L5-S1 breaks down prematurely, there is a somewhat higher chance that L4-5 could break down. If both L5-S1 and L4-L5 have degenerated, there is a higher chance that L3-4 could break down if the patient undergoes an L4-S1 fusion and does not restrict their activity.

Iliac Crest Bone Grafting

Taking an iliac crest graft was normally one of the mainstays of performing a fusion. There is a location on the back of the pelvis where there is extra bone that is not necessary for structural support. It can be accessed by a small incision or by an extension of the back incision. This bone taken is highly beneficial to generate new bone formation, essential for forming a fusion. There is some downside for taking this bone. It can leave a defect in the pelvis if not filled in with bone substitute as the muscles attach here. Sometimes, these muscular insertions develop pain, much like a tennis elbow. Occasionally, bone pain can develop, which is dull and achy. It may not be uncomfortable but, if painful, may take up to a year for this graft site pain to diminish.

Bone Morphogenic Protein (BMP)

In the last five years, we have unlocked some of the secrets of how fractured bone heals. It turns out that bone healing is really a cascade of events, just like blood clotting or inflammation. When the bone breaks, proteins are exposed that induces the healing cascade. The discovery of the makeup of some of these proteins has advanced fusion success substantially. Bone morphogenic protein (BMP) causes the body's naturally occurring stem cells to turn into bone cells. This causes faster and denser bone formation when used in a fusion.

There are some potential risks. An area of swollen tissue can occur around the BMP, causing nerve irritation; and occasionally, the BMP can erode some of the native bone, causing cavity formation before finally inducing healing.

Pseudoarthrosis

Anytime a fusion is undertaken, the potential exists for the two bones not to fuse together. This is called a pseudoarthrosis. Although many times painful, interestingly, there are times this condition may not cause symptoms. If painful, a revision surgery may need to be undertaken.

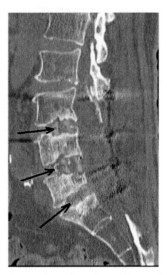

19-8—3 level pseudoarthrosis performed at another
institution—arrows point to gaps in the vertebra
that should have solid bone formation.

Recovery from Fusion

Well, now that you have undergone lumbar fusion, what can you expect from
rehabilitation? The first one to three weeks after surgery can occasionally be
challenging. Some individuals feel like they had been kicked in the back by a mule.
Other patients have minimal discomfort. The appropriate pain medications will help
through this period.

During the first three months after fusion surgery, significant restrictions in motion
of the lower back are mandatory. Limited motion will allow the bone cells to form
across the fusion site. Theoretically, increased back motion can thwart those cells from
forming a bond. Simple movements are not detrimental and probably are helpful in
promoting healing. There should be no BLT—bending, lifting, and twisting—lifting
no more than ten pounds.

The patient can and should be encouraged to do aerobic exercises. This does
not mean jogging or the weight room, but walking outside or on a treadmill, using
a stationary bike as long as the handlebars are upright and even using an elliptical
trainer, without using the arm attachment (this causes rotation). Aerobic standing
and walking pool work in a warm pool is encouraged but not actual swimming as this
causes extension and rotation.

Isometric strengthening can be performed immediately after surgery. Isometrics
pit opposing or antagonistic muscles against each other at the same time. This means
that the joints involved do not move, valuable after fusion surgery. To give an example,
if you were to contract the biceps and triceps at the same time, the elbow joint would

not move, but the two muscles would be developing strong contractions and, therefore, developing strength and conditioning.

Driving can be done as soon as the patient is not narcotized from too much medication, can sit comfortably, and can make a panic stop (you would not want to hit a child who ran in front of the car). An automatic transmission is mandatory for the first four to six weeks.

After the first six weeks, physical therapy can be instituted. This is for building endurance and isometric strengthening. Again, lumbar range of motion and activities that strain the spine need to be avoided, but PT helps to guide the patient during the healing process.

Aspirin-type medication needs to be avoided for the first three months. This group includes NSAIDs such as Motrin and Naprosyn. Aspirin-type products retard inflammation that is necessary for bone healing. Tylenol is fine to take as it is not in this category.

At the three-month point is when the patient can be encouraged to start active and passive lumbar spine range of motion exercises. Motrin and its cousins can be taken now. By the six-month point, the patient should have a solid fusion and be able to load their spine normally.

The permanent restrictions to the patient's activity depend upon their job, social activities, and the nature of their remaining discs. A patient with one-level fusion could go back to any activities. A two-level fusion could go back to the weight room and cycling but would have to reduce skiing, snowboarding, and avoid running.

Smoking and Fusion

Many times, patients ask if there is any supplement that can be taken to speed up or help the healing process. The answer is sadly no. There is, however, a chemical that has significant deleterious effects to the bone cells, and that substance is nicotine. Exposure to cigarette smoke or chew will reduce the chance of fusion by as much as 30%.

Artificial Discs

These sound like a good idea. We have implanted artificial joints for the knees and hips for a number of years, and they work very well. An artificial disc makes sense. To keep motion preserved sounds like a good idea. There are, however, significant differences between replacing knee and hip joints and replacing discs.

The reason that joint replacement works so well is the anatomical location of the joint. They are superficial and are surrounded by only muscle and bone. This means they are easy to get to if an artificial joint goes bad or wears out. Most replacement joints fail by ten to fifteen years because of the body's reaction to the wear debris from the joint.

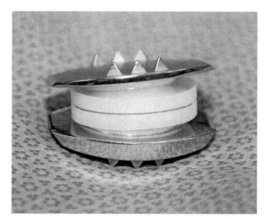

19-9 Lumbar total disc arthroplasty implant—note the plastic
sandwiched between the two metal endplates

An artificial joint is a metal surface that joins to a plastic surface. There is very little friction between the two surfaces, but there is some. The metal eventually wears the plastic surface down and the small particles that form simulate a foreign body reaction. White blood cells come in to try and "swallow" these foreign plastic "invaders" but can't digest them. These white blood cells literally burst open. The enzymes in these cells then are flushed into the local environment and start to erode the native bone away. Granulomas form, which are large clusters of WBCs and do the same thing. This eventually erodes enough bone to loosen the implant, and pain develops. The answer in the hip or knee is to make an incision, remove the debris, replace the joint with a larger one that fits into the defect, and the process starts anew.

This same action will probably occur in artificial discs. This problem could create significant complications. First, the surrounding vertebral body is eroded away, and this creates a bone deficit that can't be easily fixed like a knee replacement can. The second problem is that the inflammatory mass that surrounds the worn disc may adhere to everything. This is called a granuloma. The structures around the disc are the vena cava (the large vein that returns blood to the heart) and the aorta (the artery that brings blood to the pelvis and legs from the heart). One can imagine that having adhesions attached to these structures would make replacing a worn artificial disc difficult and possibly risky. Also, the spinal nerves are at the back of this disc, and any granulomas or erosions wouldn't be very good for this area.

A third consideration is older age. As we get older, our bones get softer. This occurs in women faster than men (osteoporosis). Normally, everything in the spine tends to adjust to this softening. What happens when the spinal bones get softer but the metal artificial disc end plate does not? A fracture of the bone would ensue, and the disc replacement may not function.

Younger age of the patient may have significant repercussions to the longevity of the implant. We try not to put a total joint replacement in young individuals as we know the prosthesis will wear them out, and a new replacement will be needed. There are only so many replacements that can be made before the bone is so worn out making further replacement next to impossible. With exceptions, fifty to sixty years of age is considered the youngest age to have a joint replacement. Total disc replacements are, however, placed into thirty-year-olds.

So in my opinion, when the flaws are engineered out, the future will probably look good for replacement discs. The present is probably not the time to consider one. In addition, fusion works very well for the same problem that these artificial discs treat. Fusion also lasts the life of the patient. We are still some distance away from developing a disc that is reliable and has longevity.

Scoliosis and Deformity

The term "scoliosis" as noted before means an abnormal curve greater than ten degrees. Scoliosis by itself is generally not a reason to consider surgery. When does the curve need to be addressed surgically?

Curves in the lumbar spine can advance in severity. If the curve can be demonstrated to advance through serial x-rays through the years and be expected to continue to advance, then surgery for the curve is warranted.

For an adult with degenerative scoliosis, the spine can and does wear out prematurely. This means that all the typical problems that occur with a normal aging spine also occur with a scoliotic spine, but at a younger age.

Surgery for specific problems (degenerative spondylolisthesis or herniated disc) can be taken care of without addressing the scoliosis. But remember, the degenerative scoliotic spine can be like a house of cards. One area of the spine surgically managed through a decompression for leg pain can lose its tenuous stability and collapse, leading to other parts of the spine causing problems. The small amount of spur that was removed to decompress a nerve may have conferred some intrinsic stability. That is, the spur had formed to keep the spine from further collapsing. Removing the spur can lead to further collapse, causing a recompression of the nerve that was originally decompressed or causing an additional stress on an adjacent segment, leading to different symptoms.

To straighten and fuse an adult scoliotic spine requires an extensive surgery involving multiple levels. The debility of having adult degenerative scoliosis can be so severe that the surgery is warranted.

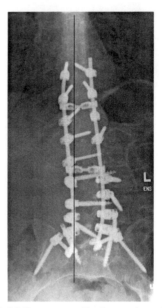

19-10 Post op scoliosis repair-rods
hold spine until fusion sets

The adolescent scoliotic spine may occasionally also need surgery, but that issue is not addressed in this book

Implantable Devices for Stenosis Treatment (Kyphogenic Devices)

There are devices made that can be inserted with a small incision that sits between the spinous processes to spread them apart. This causes the two vertebrae to permanently hold a flexion position. As noted in previous chapters, for a patient with spinal stenosis or foraminal stenosis, flexion opens the canal, which is why many patients get relief from forward flexion. This surgery is minimally invasive but has some costs to it.

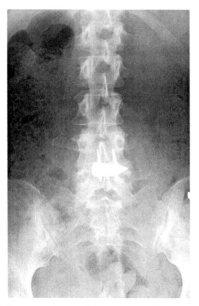

19-11 X-Stop positioned between spinous processes

First, it does not address the problem of a narrowed canal or narrowed foramen. Spending another hour of surgical time can solve that problem by doing the actual surgical decompression. Second, it causes the two vertebrae to be held in flexion. To reiterate, as we age, the discs degenerate and cause a flatter lumbar lordosis. This device aggravates that problem, but if the patient has good compensatory mechanisms, this may be a moot point. The third is that the device is made of metal or hard plastic and could cause the two spinous processes where it is wedged in between to erode or fracture.

On the plus side is that if the patient is medically unstable, a smaller surgery would be less risky and more tolerable.

Vertebroplasty and Kyphoplasty

These two procedures are designed for compression fractures in the elderly. They were previously covered in the chapter on osteoporosis. Essentially, both are designed to stabilize the fractured vertebra by injecting cement into the damaged body. This does confer immediate stability as the cement sets in minutes. The drawback is that even though the cement stabilizes the fracture, it prevents healing of the fractured fragments. In addition, the cement is harder than the surrounding vertebra and can act as a stress riser to allow fracture of adjacent vertebra.

Failed Surgery Syndrome

There is a group of patients that undergo surgery, and they have results that are not satisfactory. These patients may have had a surgical failure for reasons not yet defined. Any patient who has undergone a fusion may have developed a pseudoarthrosis. This is a failure of the intended vertebrae to fuse together and can be diagnosed with appropriate studies. Patients with continued leg pain may have had incomplete decompression, recurrent decompression, or a collapse of the surgical area and new onset compression. This can also be diagnosed with care. Rarely, the diagnosis that led to the surgery could have been faulty, leading to an incorrect surgical procedure.

Many of the failed procedures can be improved somewhat or greatly with the correct diagnostic workup and appropriate surgical procedures.

20

How to Pick a Good-Treating Health Care Provider

There are many types and abilities of providers to pick from when contemplating care of your back pain. This chapter will help to guide you through the complex world of choices. The end of this section will list the specifics of training that these experts have to meet before they can call themselves by a title such as physical therapist, chiropractor, spine surgeon, etc. First, it is a good idea to know what skill sets are needed for the providers you meet.

Skill Sets for Any Treating Providers

There are some basic foundations that can provide an understanding of the problem and then the development of an effective treatment program. These basics are built on an underpinning of compassion, understanding, and completeness.

The basics are the caregiver's knowledge of differential diagnosis and physical examination, the ability to know when to order and how to interpret further tests, the ability to educate the patient about the disorder, the ability to have the best referral medical personnel or therapists to help treat the patient, and, finally, if the choice is a surgeon, the ability to be an outstanding and meticulous surgeon. Patient satisfaction obviously hinges on good outcomes to treatment.

Differential Diagnosis

Knowledge of differential diagnosis is important. The famous Harvard physician Dr. William Osler made an astute observation that most physicians live by. "You see what you know, and you find what you look for." In other words, you have to know what can go wrong to identify it, and you have to look for it, or you won't find it if it is present. The caregiver has to know the spectrum of what causes pain or symptoms and how to identify it. This defines both the science and *the art* of medicine.

A patient can present with leg pain. The differential can include nerve pain, muscle pain, referral (sclerotomal) pain, spinal cord pain, and even poor circulation or a blood clot. If the physician doesn't think of the possibility of a blood clot, this could be a significant error. Even if the therapist had never had the experience of seeing a particular disorder, but has digested a significant amount of literature, he or she will be prepared to identify it. A physician has to be "on their toes" to be aware of possible misleading symptoms and have a good differential diagnosis.

Diagnostic proficiency comes through experience and a thorough history and physical examination. A complete history of the problems is essential. Any family history of back disorders or even of non-spine-related issues such as ulcerative colitis? Some back problems stem from related diseases and may need to be treated differently. Psoriasis (a common skin disorder) has associated spinal problems and has a different treatment protocol. It is also important to discover if there are any legal issues such as automobile accidents or work history and who may be at fault. Legal issues can shade results of the history and need special types of treatment.

A good review of the individual's general health is important. Through a good history and nothing else, 80% of the diagnoses of low back and leg pain can be ascertained.

Physical Examination

The physical exam needs to be complete, and the skill of the examiner is very important. There are some very subtle "shades of gray" that can shed light between various disorders. The diagnostician may need to identify the difference between a plus-2 and a plus-1 reflex, sometimes a slight difference, but this may give an important clue to the cause of the pain. The skill to perform a great exam takes experience, attention to detail, and time. The examiner needs to be thorough.

A patient just came into the office that had leg pain and aching for six weeks. This patient also happened to be a chiropractor as was thinking nerve pain as we also assumed by the symptoms. Some parts of the exam demonstrated possible nerve root pain, but the patient also had no pulse in the affected leg! It turns out he had a blood clot in the artery in his leg. A simple matter of not being thorough and checking pulses would have missed this very important diagnosis.

Confirmatory Testing

The second skill set is the ability to decide what further tests (if any) would be applicable to complement and confirm the initial impression (presumed diagnosis). Not just the ability to order the right tests but the ability to thoroughly interpret these test results is important. Occasionally, the interpreter (for example, a radiologist), not knowing all the clinical information, may not know how to interpret the results. Some of the information gleaned from the tests can lie in a gray area. The investigations that image the spine are x-rays, MRIs, CT scans, bone scans, tomograms, myelograms, and

SPECT scans. Tests like EMGs that look at nerve function can be helpful in shedding some light on the diagnosis.

Education

The third skill necessary and most important is taking the care and responsibility to educate the patient about their basic illness. Patients need to have the information demystified in a manner that is basic and understandable. This knowledge must be conveyed to the patient in a comprehendible manner with visual aids if necessary. If a patient cannot understand and grasp the problem, then the treatment will be less effective, and the patient's expectations for success will be murky. The mystery and fear of disabling low back pain can be significant. Education removes this mystery and eliminates fear of the unknown.

Treatment Protocol Technique

The fourth skill of a caregiver is the art and ability to develop a treatment protocol that is reasonable, effective, and appropriate for the patient. This cannot be a cookbook technique. The approach and even the personality of the therapist and patient have to be taken into consideration. This may include different types of physical therapy, chiropractic, activity modification, medication, injection, alternative therapy, massage, and even surgery when needed. Treatment needs to be cost effective as medical care is very expensive and escalating yearly. The knowledge of well-qualified specialists to refer to for further diagnostic testing or treatment is important. A good spine expert can often be like a quarterback. He or she looks at the defense (diagnosis), calls the plays (treatment), and then passes or hands off to another health care provider for the necessary tests or care.

Picking Which Provider to Trust

So who do you go to? There are as many choices as there are colors in the rainbow.

There are a number of distinct physicians within the medical world (including medical doctors and doctors of osteopathy) that you have a choice from. Internists, family physicians, orthopaedists, neurosurgeons, spine surgeons, physical medicine and rehabilitation specialists, neurologists, anesthesiologists, and even some psychiatrists that treat lower back disorders. There are places that have multiple specialists who treat these disorders as a group.

There are many types of nonmedical practitioners to choose from, and they vary greatly even within their own specialty. You can go to a chiropractor, physical therapist, massage therapist, athletic trainer, acupuncturist, Feldenkrais or Pilates practitioner, personal trainer, athletic trainer, or even an aroma therapist.

Internists and Family Practice Physicians

Internists and family physicians are the most typical entry into the world of medical treatment. The second most common reason for a visit to your primary care doctor is back pain. These individuals have one of the most difficult jobs. These doctors have to know about heart disease, circulation, lungs, liver, kidney, diabetes, infectious disease, as well as the spine. They have the hardest job in medicine.

These docs might initially use medications and activity restrictions. If their treatment is not effective, they might refer to a physical therapist. Some may refer to chiropractors. Osteopaths may treat the problem themselves with manipulation and muscle techniques. No matter to which you go, if the problem is resolved, obviously there is no further need of treatment.

Physician Specialists

The **physical medicine and rehabilitation (PM&R)** doctor has a four-year residency after medical school that is different from the orthopaedist, spine surgeon, or neurosurgeon. They are not surgeons and are given a comprehensive education in spinal disorders. These doctors can specialize in nonsurgical treatment of the back. Many perform EMGs that are electrical nerve diagnostic tests to help understand the source of nerve pain. Others have taken fellowships in interventional spinal injections to complement their treatment programs. These individuals are a good choice for initial treatment.

The **neurologist** also can have an excellent understanding of spinal disorders. They have a four-year post-medical school residency. Most specialize in the diagnosis and treatment of neurological disorders of which spinal disorders are a component. Some can have extensive training in spinal biomechanics, and many gain this knowledge in their practice. They are the true experts in diagnosing specific nerve disorders such as peripheral neuropathy and multiple sclerosis. They specialize in EMGs. Most times, you would be referred to this specialist by your family doctor or specialist.

The **rheumatologist** is another choice as a treating physician. He or she is a specialist in joint disorders that include the spine. They first do a residency in internal medicine and then do a fellowship in rheumatology. These are the true specialists in autoimmune joint disorders such as rheumatoid arthritis and SLE (lupus) among others. Again, you normally would see this specialist by referral from another physician.

Doctors of osteopathy are probable one of the most misunderstood of all the physician groups. They are trained in anatomy, physiology, and pathology in osteopathic schools exactly the same as in medical schools. After graduation, many take residencies in the medical world, and some take osteopathic residencies. In general, they are essentially medical doctors with the initials DO (doctor of osteopathy) instead of MD. All are trained in osteopathic manipulation, but many don't use this form of therapy in their practice. Many are specialists after taking a residency such as PM&R, neurology, or orthopaedics. Many are a good first choice for back care.

Chiropractic

The chiropractor spends four academic years after college to gain their doctorate degree in chiropractic. The chiropractic college is separate and distinct from the medical schools. This education follows somewhat the medical school model for the first two years including cadaver dissection, physiology, and pathology. The education differs from the traditional allopathic model in that they also learn biomechanics, manipulation of the spine (the chiropractic adjustment), and physical therapy modalities. Herbal and diet therapies accompany their education. After four academic years, he or she must pass the national and state boards and then open their own private practice. Chiropractors can diagnose and treat many spinal disorders and are trained in x-ray usage and understanding to augment their diagnosis.

Some chiropractors take a postgraduate degree. The specialities include orthopaedics, neurology, sports medicine, and even internal medicine. Chiropractors do not have prescriptive medication rights and, therefore, cannot write for medications. The mainstay of chiropractic treatment is the manipulation of spinal segments. For patients with restriction of motion, this treatment can be very effective. Many utilize rehabilitation procedures to augment their manipulation skills, and education is important.

Most mainstream chiropractors pursue the modern diagnostic systems. Following the typical degenerative cascade that occurs in many individuals, there is asymmetric and faulty motion that occurs in the vertebral segments. This restriction of motion can cause adhesions, compensatory muscle straining, and "capsular catching" of the lining of the facet joints. The "adjustment" used by chiropractors breaks the vacuum seal of the facet joint. This causes the distinctive "pop" heard and felt by the patient. This move allows increased motion that may give significant relief of pain. Muscle spasm may also be relieved by this maneuver.

Using office and home exercise, a chiropractor will attempt to increase the spine's motion and strength. Modalities such as heat, ultrasound, electrical muscle stimulation, and massage are used to relax the patient and help with muscle spasm.

Some chiropractors still believe that misalignments of the spine cause disease and treat the spine as the source of many other disorders. These chiropractors are a special subset and won't be discussed in this book.

Physical Therapy

The physical therapist spends four to six years in college before getting a bachelor's or master's degree in PT. These individuals are very well trained in anatomy, biomechanics, and exercise therapy. They have therapeutic machines at their disposal to reduce swelling and promote healing. Some therapists strictly specialize in spinal rehabilitation, and others are generalists, treating all joints in the body as well as stroke patients and cardiac rehabilitation.

They are the experts in looking at the body for injuries and developing a treatment protocol to help heal and compensate for injury. They are the mainstays for many physicians to treat the lumbar spine.

Personal Trainers

If personal trainers have been through an athletic training degree, they are the normally well educated about the body. They have not had formal diagnosis courses, but if something is painful, most will avoid that activity. Many are great at core training, the training of the muscles around your "core."

Surgeons

Some surgeons may be a good choice as primary caregivers. Surgeons are thought of as performing only surgery, but that is generally not the case. There are some surgeons that only perform surgery and will only see a patient upon referral from a primary doctor. However, there are many great diagnostitions that have good conservative treatment guidelines. Only the rare surgeon has the surgical philosophy: "If all I have is a hammer, the whole world looks like a nail." Seek their counsel if you are only considering the surgical option. There are many ways to treat spinal disorders, and most of the time, surgery is only one of many options.

Orthopaedic Surgeons

The orthopaedist is a surgeon and is formally trained for five years in a residency after four years in medical school. He or she is trained to treat all types of neurological and bony disorders, both surgically and nonsurgically. A good portion of this time is spent with spinal disorders. Most of these individuals have a very good understanding of the biomechanics and biochemical nature of the spine and can design a good treatment program. Many, however, are becoming more specialized in specific treatment areas such as the knee or shoulder and refraining from treating spinal disorders.

Spine Surgeons

The spine surgeon is an orthopaedist who has taken an additional fellowship with a recognized program specifically to treat spinal disorders for an extra year after finishing the five-year orthopaedic residency. These individuals generally have an excellent understanding of the conservative and surgical treatment of the spine. Most only treat spinal disorders.

Neurosurgeons

The neurosurgeon completes a surgical residency in neurosurgery that takes six years. They spend a good portion of their time with spinal disorders, and many are the equivalent of the spine surgeon in knowledge and understanding. Some neurosurgeons don't treat the spine, but perform brain surgery only. Some neurosurgeons take spine fellowships to increase their scope.

Should I Go to a Spine Surgeon or a Neurosurgeon?

Today, there are very few differences between spine surgeons and neurosurgeons in regard to the spine and spine care. In the past, differences were more substantial. The orthopaedic spine surgeons come from a background of scoliosis and spine reconstruction, spinal fusion for instability. Neurosurgeons come from the tumor/decompression side. Over the last ten years, the lines have been blurred, and in reality, there is minimal difference. Again, in my opinion, it is the surgeon himself or herself that makes the difference and not necessarily if he or she is a spine surgeon or neurosurgeon. About the only differences today are that most spine surgeons don't resect tumors in the spinal cord, and most neurosurgeons don't perform scoliosis surgery.

As you can see, there is an incredible number of different types of caregivers that can help you out of pain. How you choose them has to do with their education, specialty, reputation, the personal interactions you have with them, and your final satisfaction.

Index